Translation and Health Risk Knowledge Building in China

Meng Ji

Translation and Health Risk Knowledge Building in China

palgrave
macmillan

Meng Ji
The University of Sydney
Sydney, NSW
Australia

ISBN 978-981-10-4680-3   ISBN 978-981-10-4681-0 (Ebook)
DOI 10.1007/978-981-10-4681-0

Library of Congress Control Number: 2017939555

© The Editor(s) (if applicable) and The Author(s) 2017
This work is subject to copyright. All rights are solely and exclusively licensed by the Publisher, whether the whole or part of the material is concerned, specifically the rights of translation, reprinting, reuse of illustrations, recitation, broadcasting, reproduction on microfilms or in any other physical way, and transmission or information storage and retrieval, electronic adaptation, computer software, or by similar or dissimilar methodology now known or hereafter developed.
The use of general descriptive names, registered names, trademarks, service marks, etc. in this publication does not imply, even in the absence of a specific statement, that such names are exempt from the relevant protective laws and regulations and therefore free for general use.
The publisher, the authors and the editors are safe to assume that the advice and information in this book are believed to be true and accurate at the date of publication. Neither the publisher nor the authors or the editors give a warranty, express or implied, with respect to the material contained herein or for any errors or omissions that may have been made. The publisher remains neutral with regard to jurisdictional claims in published maps and institutional affiliations.

Cover illustration: © saulgranda/Getty

Printed on acid-free paper

This Palgrave Macmillan imprint is published by Springer Nature
The registered company is Springer Nature Singapore Pte Ltd.
The registered company address is: 152 Beach Road, #21-01/04 Gateway East, Singapore 189721, Singapore

ACKNOWLEDGEMENT

This study is supported by of a Discovery Project (DP150102405) funded by the Australian Research Council (2015–2018). It involves the collaboration of major translation research centres in Europe, Australia, North America and Brazil: University of Ghent, Belgium; University College London; University of Bari, Italy; Federal University of Minas Gerais, Brazil; Kent State University, USA, with The University of Sydney as the lead university on this project.

CONTENTS

LIST OF FIGURES

LIST OF TABLES

CHAPTER 1

Introduction

Abstract Translation of health policy represents a critical yet largely underexplored research area. This book offers an empirical corpus linguistic analysis of the translation and the dissemination of global health policies in China, focusing on the linguistic translation and cultural adaptation of terms and expressions of public health financial risks and social welfare system reform in official materials developed by authoritative international health agencies like the World Health Organisation.

Keywords Chinese translation studies · Health translation · Corpus linguistics

Rapid advances in information technologies such as natural language processing and more recently, statistical machine translation tools have significantly changed the landscape of scientific and health translation. Translation Studies emerged as a rapidly evolving field of research which lies at the crossroad of social sciences, humanities and information science. The current study of the translation, variation and cultural assimilation of health financial risk terms deploy empirical research methodologies widely used in corpus translation studies, which is one of the most dynamic research areas of contemporary translation studies. The translation phenomenon investigated in this book is the conceptual and formal variation of health financial risk terminologies in translation. In this book, variant translations of healthcare financial risks terms are defined as linguistic expressions used by different translators in the target culture and society. These culturally localised translations cannot be treated as conventional linguistic synonyms in the target language. By contrast, the corpus analysis shows that localised health translations tend to exhibit levels of conceptual and formal variations of the original English health terminologies. This can be examined in the use of these expressions in the Chinese formal discourses, for example, by looking at the distinct collocation patterns of the translated terms in large-scale databases of Chinese research publications, as well as their contrastive distributions across research disciplines of the target knowledge system.

This study argues that the wide existence of translation terminological variation of health financial risk terms in Chinese public health materials reflects the largely developing nature of the public health knowledge system in the country. It mirrors the cross-cultural communication process in the early stages of the introduction and translation of modern western sciences in China in the late nineteenth century. The establishment of a consistent scientific terminology system played an instrumental role in the development of modern sciences in China at the turn of the twentieth century. Amidst intensified historical cross-cultural and cross-lingual interactions, a large number of translated scientific terms were created and used by different translators in an effort to bridge significant conceptual and cultural gaps between the source and the target languages.

Science translation has provided a focus of significant research in the study of science history and modernisation in China both inside and outside of the country. In the process of cross-cultural and cross-lingual contact and interaction, the co-existence and competition for standardisation and conventionalisation in the target language between different translation approaches and schools was well documented. Terminological variability reflects the developing nature of the Chinese science language, and the ongoing cultural and social transition and the establishment of modern sciences in the country.

This study argues that an important factor in the social or cultural selection and the establishment of new translated terms is the dissemination and cultural acceptance of particular translation options by the target audience. In early historical periods, the dissemination of translated materials was largely restricted to social and economic elites. The general public had restricted access to and knowledge of translated materials. That is, in these historical periods, the chief social function of translation was to provide referential materials for the administration and governing social groups, rather than inform the public.

With increasing cross-cultural communication and rapid advances in natural language processing and machine learning technologies since the mid-twentieth century, translation has become an integral part of the everyday social life in many parts of the world, especially in developing countries where new scientific knowledge systems evolve at a level and speed rarely seen before. The study of the social functions of science translation which is instrumental to the ongoing process of globalisation has been given increased visibility and importance. This study is embedded within this larger social and cultural context. It intends to make useful efforts to explore the interaction and interplay between different approaches to cross-lingual and cross-cultural health research translation in general, and the development of public understanding and knowledge around healthcare financial risks in particular.

The book maintains that the translation of health policy materials requires an in-depth understanding of the existing cultural conventions and accepted communication styles in the target language and society. The empirical analysis in this book using both original longitudinal and contrastive (English and Chinese) linguistic databases suggests that health translation strategies should include first of all, an adequate cultural adaptation of health materials which highlights the consistencies and links between the source and the target health knowledge systems and social practices; secondly, effective cross-lingual translation methods which utilise and exploit typical linguistic resources of the target language such as conventionalised syntactic and lexicographical constructs—serving as *translation moulds*—in the creation of new health terminologies. This proposed highly skilful translation and purposeful language transformation approach stands in contrast with the literal translation, i.e. translation word by word, and the heavily domesticated translation strategy. Neither of these two somewhat polarised methods can fulfil the important social and communicative function of health translation which is to deliver research-intensive knowledge and information in a responsible and effective way. The corpus analysis shows that health translations which were produced in line with such translation principles tend to be better understood, accepted and widely disseminated in the target language and culture.

A methodological innovation of this book is that it integrates both textual and contextual or social analyses in the corpus-based study of health translations. Translation Studies have long been divided between the two distinct sets of research agendas, i.e. micro-linguistic and macro-social translation studies. In this book, the detailed systematic linguistic analysis of health policy translation is first of all, preceded by a review of the social and cultural contexts in which healthcare reforms and policy research was introduced and carried out in China, and then followed by a quantitative and statistical modelling of the dissemination of newly introduced health risk concepts and knowledge in the target culture and society.

This book has significantly advanced a research area which has received little attention and has been explored to a very limited extent in Chinese translation studies. Specifically, this book suggests that the social selection and cultural acceptance of particular translations over other translation possibilities—which form part of the so-called translation variation in this study—can be measured and studied by comparing the statistical indicators provided by large-scale databases of Chinese formal publications. A longitudinal analysis revealed the shifting focus and varying levels of interest in specific health topics among researchers, media professionals and the general public in China. By leveraging and integrating well-established research methodologies from information science, corpus linguistics and textual statistics, this book aims to explore new lines of research for corpus cross-lingual health translation. It represents a useful effort to advance latest empirical translation studies and to bring much-needed insights into the social role and function of the translation of health policy and research in a globalised contemporary world.

This study examines the development of health policy knowledge in China at an early stage of health policy translation in China, i.e. around the late 1990s and the early 2000s which was before the advent of the wide use of machine translation software such as web-based statistical translation tools like Google Translate and cloud translation terminology databases. It offers an empirical corpus analysis of different attempts and efforts made by translators to interpret and culturally contextualise English health risks terms in a typologically different language, Mandarin Chinese. Health translation entails the linguistic remoulding and shaping of the Chinese health policy language, and more importantly, the introduction and establishment of new concepts and idea sets of global health policy research in the native cultural and knowledge system.

The focus of the linguistic analysis is to identify and compare the different translation strategies that have been experimented within such an important process, instead of passing on a subjective judgement or criticism between good and bad translations, as health policy translation requires the combination of a range of highly specialised expertise and skills. The terminological variation detected in health policy translation points to the need and urgency of systematic research in this area, as well as possible directions for developing efficient and effective methodologies for the translation of global health policy as a field of growing social and research significance.

The proliferation of variant translations, the corpus analysis shows, is a wide-existing phenomenon in intensified cross-cultural and cross-lingual science interactions. The detected variation and variability of health translation terminology reflects the dynamics of the conceptual and language alignment between the source and the target societies and systems of knowledge. Different from text-based translation studies that tend to be qualitative and rely on limited case studies, the corpus-based approach to translation studies takes full advantage of the availability of large-scale digital resources and related corpus mining technologies and tools. The technical convenience afforded by monolingual and multilingual digital resources and tools can greatly facilitate the empirical analysis of health translation variation. This helps researchers to develop new translation evaluation methods which are fundamentally based on the cultural and linguistic acceptance and use of the translated concepts and terms among the target audiences. This book explains and illustrates this end-user-oriented research agenda which can be achieved through the integration of statistical analyses and modelling techniques in the empirical study of health translation materials.

The combination of methodologies used in corpus translation studies and data mining techniques can assist researchers of translation studies in the development of empirical measures and instruments to extract and analyse underlying patterns of the distribution and dissemination of translation materials. The methodologies developed in this book, particularly in Chaps. 4 and 5, draw upon the well-tested corpus linguistic methodologies. The corpus study will fill in the long-existing gap in the study of the impact of translation on the development of health risks knowledge in the target language, culture and science knowledge system.

By using public health translation as a case study, this book illustrates the feasibility and productivity of integrating a range of interdisciplinary research methodologies for the study of health translation. For example, the use of corpus materials and corpus methodologies can effectively detect subtle yet important differences in variant health translations of key public health concepts. The combination of translation methods with data mining techniques can help to develop measurements to analyse the patterns of the growth and dissemination of health risk knowledge in the target society and culture, as influenced by translations. Again, the adaptation and integration of research methodologies across disciplines from linguistics, translation studies, statistics and comparative social and cultural studies lies at the very heart of the original research efforts and contributions made in this book to advance global health policy translation.

This book is divided into seven chapters. Chapter 2 outlines the study of health risk translation as a new research area and efforts made by this study to fill in a gap of knowledge in this critical research area. Chapter 3 provides a brief review of the development of the healthcare and social security system in China, and the use of specific public health terms and expressions in different historical periods in the country. English translations of selected original Chinese health materials are provided to demonstrate the features and characteristics of the developing Chinese healthcare system since the mid-twentieth century. The extraction of Chinese research resources was through using the keyword search function (yī liáo bǎo xiǎn zhì dù or healthcare system) to explore the largest publication database in China, the Chinese Knowledge Resources Integrated Network also known as CNKI.

To facilitate understanding of the parallel growth of the international and native Chinese public health policy research, Chap. 3 provides the social and contextual background to the translation and introduction of public health risk terms in official documents of the WHO in China in the 1990s. In Chap. 3, discussions on the Chinese health research context and the international health research environment are developed using keyword analysis of Chinese and English publications, a research method which is widely used in corpus linguistics and corpus translation studies.

Chapter 4 introduces the construction of a parallel English-Chinese corpus of WHO health translations. It gives details of the practical consideration in the collection of corpus materials to build the parallel corpus. The construction of the parallel corpus facilitates the identification and extraction of English health risk terms which gave rise to competing translations or the detected terminological variation in health translation, the translation phenomenon which is highlighted in this chapter and discussed at length in this book. The variant translations extracted in the parallel corpus exploration were grouped into different clusters of health risk terminologies that underscored the development and building of new health risks knowledge among the target audiences.

The conceptually defined clusters of health terminologies were used in the following chapter for the corpus analysis of the semantic and usage differences between variant translations of imported health risk terms and concepts. The linguistic analysis of parallel corpora of original English texts and their Chinese versions revealed that semantic and terminological variability, as indicated by variant translations, widely exists in health financial risk translation. This reflects a critical gap in current health translation practice and research. The corpus analyses found that among variant health translations within the same conceptual cluster, some were new expressions developed on the basis of the English source texts; and some linguistic expressions had strong linguistic and cultural roots in the target Chinese language.

Chapter 5 deploys large Chinese databases to analyse the collocation and disciplinary distribution patterns of variant translations of health terms in Chinese research publications. The corpus-based longitudinal analysis compares over an extended period of time newly created health expressions with health translations adapted from or simply borrowing existing culturally conventionalised terms in Chinese formal discourses. The corpus-based empirical analysis suggests that culturally and linguistically localised expressions of health financial risks tend to be better construed and established in the target Chinese knowledge system. The corpus analysis of variant health risk translations also reveals that the focus and specific approaches to critical health topics such as healthcare financial risks exhibit different patterns at the international and national levels. This book makes a useful effort to discuss and analyse this important social and research issue from the perspective of quantitative translation studies as a rapidly developing field of empirical translation studies which came to the fore in the early 2000s.

Chapter 6 provides a corpus-based exploration of the distribution of health translations using a trend analysis and the subsequent statistical modelling of variant health translations in Chinese research publication. It was found that health terms which form the culturally adapted translation group occurred much more frequently in Chinese research publications, when compared to entirely newly created translations or word-by-word literal translations without adequate cultural and linguistic adaptation. It was interesting to notice that in some cases, despite temporal decrease in the frequency of occurrence of certain culturally rooted and linguistically remoulded translations in the databases, often as result of the introduction of new translations in certain periods of time and a surge in public interest in specific health topics triggered by social events and the media, the temporary decrease of such translations may be reversed over a larger timespan. This is a corpus-based finding which again testifies to the importance of developing and establishing culturally and linguistically appropriate health policy translation systems and strategies.

Chapter 6 utilised the statistical measures produced by large-scale databases to develop useful indicators for the study of the patterns of the distribution of health translation variants in the target language and social context. These indicators can furnish a set of useful measures to gauge the social impact and significance of health translation materials in the target cultural and knowledge environment. The research findings presented in this chapter thus yield useful insights into the process through which the purposeful use of translation methods and techniques may affect the academic dissemination rate (ADR) and media dissemination rate (MDR) of the original source materials in the targeted health research environment. These two indicators, i.e. ADR and MDR, may in turn collectively influence the rate of growth and the patterns of information dissemination, in this case, healthcare financial risk knowledge in the Chinese society as measured by the statistical indicator of academic growth rate (AGR).

CHAPTER 2

Health Translation and Construction of Public Health Risk Knowledge

Abstract Health financial risk is a critical research and social issue in a large part of the world. Yet the linguistic translation and cultural interpretation of health financial risks represent a largely underexplored area of research. This study offers an empirical linguistic analysis of Chinese translations of global public health policy by authoritative international health agencies like the World Health Organisation. The current study intends to move away from the traditional emphasis of translation studies on the linguistic equivalence between the source and target texts, to the corpus empirical analysis of the phenomenon of translation variability, i.e. the co-existence of different possibilities of health terminological translation.

Keywords Health translation · Corpus linguistics
World Health Organisation

Latest statistics show that three-quarters of the world's population are non-native English speakers (Neeley 2012). Translation, which entails the transfer of information across languages and cultures, plays a critical role in the dissemination of public health knowledge and international policy guidelines (Straus et al. 2013). How important research findings and policy guidelines on health financial risks such as those provided by the WHO are translated into different languages and subsequently construed by national audiences remains unanswered or have been explored

© The Author(s) 2017
M. Ji, *Translation and Health Risk Knowledge Building in China*,
DOI 10.1007/978-981-10-4681-0_2

to a rather limited extent. How and to what extent global health risk studies have informed the development of local health knowledge systems? How do local knowledge systems grow in parallel with international health risk policy research? These are some of the key questions that will be explored in this study which represents an important effort to advance current health translation studies.

The linguistic analysis is conducted in two stages to address the research questions highlighted in this study. The first stage entails the contrastive linguistic analysis between original WHO health policy materials, such as its annual global health reports which are indicative of the focus and priorities of public health research at an international level, and the official Chinese translations of these key policy documents.[1] The linguistic analysis at this stage was essentially qualitative, as it involved detailed and thorough comparison of the different semantic meaning between the original English expressions and the Chinese translations created. The contrastive linguistic analysis helps to establish the cross-lingual links and associations, appropriately or problematically, by bilingual health workers and/or professional translators between the original English materials and the Chinese target texts.

The linguistic analysis shows that in many cases, the semantic correspondence between the English health expressions and the Chinese translations is not unique. In other words, an English word may well be adapted and matched with or translated to a number of Chinese terms which are defined out of convenience as variant translations in this book. The co-existence of variant translations seems to characterise earlier and to some extent, current public health risks translation. Would the co-existence of health terminologies hinder shared understanding of public health risks among social stakeholders including policy-makers, health professionals, businesses and the public? This is a research topic which has been explored to a very limited extent by far.

To address this question, the linguistic analysis conducted at the next stage focuses on the differences between variant translations identified in original Chinese publications. Large-scale databases of research publications and printed media materials are used to examine patterns of the distribution and use in original Chinese publications of translation variations identified in the first stage of linguistic analysis. This drew upon the use of quantitative scientific publications and printed media materials in the target language over a wide time frame. In this study, the use of the Chinese Knowledge Sources Integrated Network, also known as the

CNKI database enabled the statistical analysis and modelling of the distribution of variant translations in Chinese publications between as early as the 1910s until the present day.

It was found that translations which represent important local linguistic variants co-exist and compete with translations newly introduced from international health documents. In translation studies, these health translations identified point to two sets of underlying translation principles and tactics that are known as domestication and foreignisation. However, it should be pointed out that translated terms retrieved from the parallel English-Chinese corpus of WHO public health risks (details on the process of the construction of the parallel corpus are given in this chapter) exhibit mixed features that do not suggest a binary or dichotomic approach to the study of health translation. In other words, these health variant translations can be only studied in relation to each other to enable the assessment of the levels of cultural and linguistic adaptation of source language expressions in the target language.

This widely existent localisation tendency in health translation has important implications. First of all, translations which integrate linguistic and cultural elements in the target language tend to be better represented than translations that fail to do so, particularly over a long time span. For example, (see details in Chaps. 4 and 5) the term 'health financial risk factor'—originally introduced from English health policy materials—has been used to a limited extent when compared to translations such as 'dangerous factor' and 'dangerous element' which represent culturally rooted and linguistically conventionalised translation possibilities. Despite important semantic differences—risk factors, although can lead to potential loss and harms cannot be equalled with dangers—these culturally adapted expressions are often used as variant translations to the more exact translation of 'risk factor' in original Chinese scientific and media publications. The phenomenon of health translation variation points to the lack of health risk knowledge in the target health science system at the time.

The empirical analysis shows that translation variants tend to exhibit distinct collocation or lexical co-occurrence patterns that reflect their specific and subtle use in the target social, cultural and textual contexts. As a result, readers of health policy translations may unconsciously or consciously interpret these expressions in different and even contrasting manners. Without due consideration of this translation process, which is of particular relevance for the cross-cultural interpretation of health policy-making that often involves important consensus building among multisectoral stakeholders, an indiscriminative use of linguistic terms or translation variants may well mislead the reading and the subsequent construal of highly specialised source texts by the target audiences.

Secondly, few translation studies touched on the research issue of the complex process underlying the systematic cultural assimilation and uptake of translated health policy concepts and terms in the target language and society. The extent to which the translation of new health knowledge is understood by the target readership and is subsequently represented and built into the target health knowledge remains largely understudied. This has overlooked the important fact that translation is first and foremost a cross-lingual and cross-cultural communication tool; and the significance of translation, especially specialised translation of health knowledge, needs to be evaluated in terms of the social impact and uptake of the translation produced.

The research goal that has driven the design of this study is to explore different approaches to and methods of the translation of health concepts and key terminologies that can be effectively understood by the target readership and thus assimilated into the target health system to catalyse the development of new health knowledge in the target society. This research design is aided by the use of large-scale corpus resources and textual mining tools to process and analyse naturally occurring texts afforded by quantitative research publications and widely circulated media materials in the target Chinese language.

Without an in-depth study of the uptake of translated health expressions in the target language and knowledge system, it would be difficult to appreciate and assess the social impact and the relevancy of global health research and policy recommendations as perceived by distinct national audiences. The present study makes a first effort to explore this issue from a quantitative cross-lingual perspective, which is enabled by the availability of large-scale national publication databases like CNKI—the largest digital publication database in the PRC—and the statistical indicators which have been developed as part of the database to facilitate and monitor the search and retrieval of information by end-users.

A highlighted methodological contribution of this study to health translation is that it takes advantage of large-scale international and national digital publication databases including policy materials, research and media materials to investigate the process which underlines the translation, diffusion and variation of health financial risk concepts, specifically from English to Mandarin Chinese used in mainland China. The design of this empirical study represents a methodological innovation in health document translation (Harkness et al. 2008). It fills in a gap in the study of the dissemination of key health concepts and terminologies in international health policy materials via translation. This study provides an empirical study of the impact of the translation of international health policies such as those from the WHO on local societies and social sectors, e.g. the academia and media at the turn of the twentieth century.

This purposely designed corpus-driven translation study sheds new light on the complex process of the translation, dissemination, the cultural selection and linguistic variation of health knowledge by using digital bilingual (English and Chinese) and original Chinese corpora. The empirical research findings illustrate how important global health research was decoded and recoded in the translation process and eventually influenced the growth of public health knowledge at a national level. From the perspective of health translation studies, the corpus analysis identified some existing factors such as the lack of effective translation techniques which have limited or hindered the dissemination of international health research, as well as influencing and informing the public understanding of health risks in national contexts.

This study aims to advance our understanding of the complexity of the process of the language translation and cultural adaptation of health risk concepts. The empirical data analysis revealed that national health knowledge systems, in this case the PRC, grew in parallel to research by authoritative international health agencies such as the WHO. This was evidenced in the high level of use of culturally loaded translation variations when compared with health terms and expressions that were introduced and translated from international health policy-making materials without undergoing the cultural and linguistic adaption and modification process.

The current study adopts a problem-focused approach to the comparison between Chinese translation variants of English health concepts and terminologies. Firstly, bilingual publications, i.e. original WHO health resources and their translations, were used to identify conceptually linked expressions of an inputted English keyword. The bilingual term pair extraction was based on statistical algorithms that are widely used in machine translation which can identify and retrieve word pairs according to their distribution patterns in the English source and the Chinese target texts. Secondly, despite their different collocation patterns, these conceptually linked expressions or translation variants of health terms as defined in the current study were examined closely to find out the underlying health concept which was then used to label this particular group of associated Chinese translation variants.

As a result of the corpus search and grouping method, linguistic expressions of specialised health concepts within the same conceptual cluster include both translations derived from and/or modelled on culturally loaded target language expressions and conventionalised lexical constructs, and newly introduced health terms apparently without such as a cultural and linguistic translation process. These health translation variants *compete for visibility and importance* in a largely developing health knowledge system in the target culture and society.

To better understand this translation phenomenon that has been discussed extensively in descriptive translation studies (Toury 1995, 2012), in the next stage, an essentially quantitative and corpus-driven analysis was conducted to explore the patterns of the use of these linguistic synonyms or translation variants. The new analytical framework designed assisted the study of the social impact of *competing translations* which encompass both existing health concepts and newly translated and introduced health topics and research focuses in the Chinese language, cultural and knowledge system.

In this study, the corpus-driven analysis led to the development of statistical indicators which measure the performance of linguistic or translation variations forming a conceptual cluster of health knowledge. An empirical assessment instrument was developed for the study of health translation variants. The assessment tool includes three new indicators which are the academic growth rate (AGR), academic dissemination rate (ADR) and media dissemination rate (MDR) of specialised terms. The new empirical assessment tool developed in this book represents the first effort in empirical translation studies to evaluate different health translation variants in international health policy documents, particularly the English and Mandarin Chinese language combination for translation is concerned.

The first two indicators, i.e. AGR and ADR, are strongly linked with and can be deployed to measure the development of specialised scientific knowledge through the volume and growth rate of academic research and publications in large-scale original Chinese databases over specific periods of time. In the current study, AGR and ADR are used to describe the aggregation and the cross-reference of academic publications in Chinese which contain linguistic and translation variations of highlighted health concepts, i.e. health financial risks. The third empirical indicator MDR is used to gauge the level of the media dissemination of linguistic variations clustering around a specific health concept. The empirical study shows that culturally loaded linguistic and lexical expressions tend to be picked up by the media more frequently when compared to highly technical terms and less familiar health translations, despite the fact that both conventionalised linguistic expressions and newly created translated terms contribute to the development of new health concepts.

The linguistic analysis has been designed to suit the development, testing and verification of new hypotheses in the corpus data processing and modelling process. For example, it was hypothesised at the outset of the corpus analysis that linguistic expressions and translation variants may be classified into the high-performance vis-à-vis the low-performance categories of health terminologies in the target language. High-performance linguistic or translation variations should, in theory, register high scores across the three empirical indicators developed, i.e. AGR, ADR and MDR. Furthermore, despite the different sets of health financial risk terms studied, for instance, some are related to risk sharing and pooling and some are related to risk-adjusted capitation, balancing and equalisation; across these health conceptual clusters, it was hypothesised that lexical expressions and translation possibilities belonging to either the high-performance category (or showing proven high uptake in the media and scientific research publications) or the low-performance (i.e. low uptake in the media and scientific research publications) category may well share important features in terms of the patterns of their computed scores across the three empirical indicators.

For this purpose, statistical analyses were used to explore any potential relationship between these three empirical indicators in an effort to ascertain whether high-performance public health terms in publications circulated in one societal sector, e.g. the academia would necessarily report similarly high dissemination rates in another societal sector, i.e. the printed and digital media.

As the corpus analysis shows in the following chapters, health expressions labelled within the same conceptual cluster exhibit different patterns of dissemination in Chinese academic publication and media resources, and within each sector across time. This empirical finding suggests that the translation of public health documents is a sensitive process, as the choice of words may well have an impact on the reach of the international health documents translated, and their acceptance by the target readership. Such results of the corpus data analysis yield valuable and much-needed insights into the (lack) of interaction between different social sectors in the generation and dissemination of health knowledge. It points to the need for improved understanding of the limits of current health translation practice whose instrumental role in the development and dissemination of international health agencies like the WHO to national audiences remains to be fully explored and investigated.

NOTE

1. The WHO website offers both the original English materials and some selected translations of these materials into its other four official languages, i.e. Chinese, Spanish, French and Russian at http://www.who.int/publications/en/.

REFERENCES

Harkness, J., B.E. Pennell, A. Villar, N. Gebler, S. Aguilar-Gaxiola, I. Bilgen, R.C. Kessler, and T.B. Üstün. 2008. Translation procedures and translation assessment in the World Mental Health Survey Initiative. *The WHO World Mental Health Surveys: Global Perspectives on the Epidemiology of Mental Disorders*, 91–113.

Neeley, Tsedal. 2012. Global Business Speaks English. Cross-Cultural Management, May 2012 available at https://hbr.org/2012/05/global-business-speaks-english.

Straus, S., J. Tetroe, and I.D. Graham, (eds.). 2013. *Knowledge translation in health care: Moving from evidence to practice*, 31 May 2013. New York: Wiley.

Toury, Gideon. 1995. *Descriptive translation studies and beyond*. Amsterdam: John Benjamins.

Toury, Gideon. 2012. *Descriptive translation studies and beyond (revised version)*. Amsterdam: John Benjamins.

CHAPTER 3

A Brief Overview of the Development of Healthcare System in China

Abstract This chapter provides a brief review of the development of the healthcare and social security system in China, and the use of specific public health terms and expressions in different historical periods in the country. English translations of selected original Chinese health materials are provided to demonstrate the features and characteristics of the developing Chinese healthcare system since the mid-twentieth century. Discussion on the Chinese health research context and the international health research environment is developed using keyword analysis of Chinese and English publications, a research method which is widely used in corpus linguistics and corpus translation studies.

Keywords Healthcare reform · Keyword analysis
Health translation terminology

In this study, the WHO (2000) Annual Report titled *Health Systems: Improving Performance* was used to build the parallel English and Chinese translation corpus (World Health Organisation 2000 Annual Report). The primary focus and aim of the WHO (2000) Annual Report was to stimulate debates around 'how a health system should be defined in order to extend our field of concern beyond the provision of public and personal health services, and encompass other key areas of public policy that have an impact on people's health' (Brundtland, former Director-General of the WHO 2000). The report broke new ground in

© The Author(s) 2017
M. Ji, *Translation and Health Risk Knowledge Building in China*,
DOI 10.1007/978-981-10-4681-0_3

that it helped the public as well as specialised audiences like health professionals and policy-makers to understand the goals of the changing and evolving global public health system.

The report defined four key functions of public health systems including the provision of health services; the generation of human and physical resources that make service delivery possible; raising and pooling the resources used to pay for public healthcare; and, most critically, the function of stewardship which is to set and enforce the rules of the game and to provide strategic direction for all the different actors involved (WHO 2000 Annual Report, viii). In this key document, public health financial risk was highlighted as an emerging and strategically important topic for both research and enhanced social practice, especially in the developing world including China.

Health financial risk represents a very new research topic and social issue in contemporary Chinese society. During the planned economy period (1949–1979), the public health welfare system in China largely focused on disease treatment and the provision of services for disease prevention and control. In the 1980s and the 1990s, with the success of the socio-economic reforms, the public healthcare system also saw important structural changes and development. There were three main types of healthcare provisions for different social sectors and population segments divided along two factors: employment funded by public funding or not; and urban vis-à-vis rural workforce. The first type of healthcare known as *Lao Bao* (Chinese abbreviation for labour protection) was targeted at employees at state-owned companies, also known as *Guo Ying Qi Ye*.

Before 1953, *Lao Bao* was entirely covered by the central government. Between 1953 and 1969, the employee contribution to *Lao Bao* was increased to between 5 and 7% of the annual salaries. This figure continued to grow after 1969 when a flat rate of 11% of the annual income of employees at state-owned companies was required by the Ministry of Finance to be put aside for private or company-run employee welfare trusts (Lin 2013). The second type of healthcare developed in the 1980s and 1990s was for employees working for governmental departments, government-funded and state-owned enterprises to promote education, culture, scientific research, health and sports, as well as for college students. This was known as *Gong Fei Yi Liao* (healthcare provision through public funding). These were the privileged group of people in the social healthcare system under development in the People's Republic of China, as their healthcare costs were entirely covered by the government.

Lastly, the third type of the hybrid and evolving Chinese national healthcare system at the time was known as *He Zuo Yi Liao* (or the so-called cooperative or contributory healthcare), which was chiefly for the country's vast rural workforce. This healthcare sector was set up with collective and individual contributions without governmental funding support. In December 1998, one year before the public release of the WHO (2000) Annual Report on global health system reform and agenda setting, the State Council of China announced the establishment of a universal healthcare security system for urban and suburban employees which was known as *Ji Ben Yi Liao Bao Xian* or the basic healthcare (State Council of the PRC, 14 December 1998). This newly introduced universal healthcare reform significantly streamlined and replaced the previous tripartite healthcare system which had clearly privileged a few social elites and disadvantaged the majority of the population.

Within the new healthcare system, companies were obliged to contribute around 6% of the wages, and the employees were required to contribute around 2% of their total earnings to the state-run healthcare system. The basic healthcare system contains two components which were the individual accounts or the so-called *Ge Ren Zhang Hu* and the centrally managed trusts or *Tong Chou Ji Jin*. While the personal contributions were deposited in their individual accounts, up to 30% of the company contribution was put into individual accounts with the remaining parts to be managed centrally by the company-run collective trusts.

Apart from the mandatory basic healthcare contributions, companies and individuals may purchase different types of supplementary healthcare policies known in Chinese as *Bu Chong Yi Liao Bao Xian* from commercial health insurance providers. These changes were described by the WHO (2000) Annual Report as 'third-generation reforms' amidst the growing 'transformation from the communist to market-oriented economies in in China, central Europe, and the former Soviet Union'. These efforts were 'more difficult to characterize than earlier reforms, because they arise for a greater variety of reasons and include more experimentation in approach' (WHO 2000 Annual Report, p. 16).

This brief overview of the development of the basic universal healthcare system in China provides the general social and cultural context in which Chinese translators and language workers viewed and interpreted the WHO (2000) Annual Report on global healthcare. To have a better understanding of the key topics and research areas around healthcare system reforms in China from the 1980s until 1999, the year immediately before the publication of the WHO (2000) Annual Report, the largest and most comprehensive publication databases in Chinese, i.e. Chinese Knowledge Net database or the CNKI database, were used in this corpus study to search for relevant research publications (Liu 2013; Wang and Wang 2015; Li et al. 2014).

The database search using 'yi liao bao xian zhi du' (the Chinese expression for healthcare insurance system) retrieved automatically more than 2,000 Chinese research publications from more than 40 academic disciplines published during this 20-year period of time under study, i.e. in the 1980s and 1990s. Table 3.1 offers a list of the keywords extracted from these research publications on healthcare system reforms in China. The corpus extraction of keywords was largely quantitative which was based on their frequencies of occurrence in the published documents extracted. In Table 3.1, No. 31 (*1) 'yǐ yào yǎng yī' is a Chinese four-character idiom which referred to an earlier public hospital survival strategy which had its origin in the planned economy period in China in the 1950s (Fang et al. 2015).

The so-called 'drug to support doctor' practice allowed public hospitals to increase and inflate the costs of medicines prescribed to the patients. Controversial incomes from the prescription and sale of high-cost medicines to the patients were used to maintain the functioning or indeed the survival of public hospitals during the communist economy period. This widely existent practice during earlier periods received strong criticism in the subsequent medical reforms starting from the early 2000s, and has gradually been replaced by the new performance-based and market-oriented healthcare provision system which is still largely under development in the country (Shen et al. 2014; Barber et al. 2013).

The top frequency words shown in Table 3.1 provide important information of main social and research topics discussed and studied in mainland China in the two decades between 1980s and the 1990s, immediately before the publication of the WHO (2000) Annual Report. These topics point to the key dimensions of healthcare reforms in the economic and social transition period in China. In order to illustrate the use and interpretation of these keywords in the Chinese textual and social context, some representative examples were chosen from the CNKI database which contained both the original Chinese texts and their English translations. The search engine of the CNKI automatically retrieved relevant textual instances from the parallel Chinese-English corpora which form part of the database (Li 2007; Hua and Su 2003).

Table 3.1 Keywords in Chinese research publications on healthcare system (1980–1999) (CNKI source)

No.	Chinese keywords	English translation	Chinese Pinyin
1	医疗保险制度	Medical insurance system	yī liáo bǎo xiǎn zhì dù
2	改革	Reform	gǎi gé
3	军队医院	Military hospital	jūn duì yī yuàn
4	医院	Hospital	yī yuàn
5	医院管理	Hospital management	yī yuàn guǎn lǐ
6	结构调整	Structural adjustment	jié gòu tiáo zhěng
7	总量控制	Total volume control	zǒng liàng kòng zhì
8	政府	Government	Zhèng fǔ
9	社会保障制度	Social security system	shè huì bǎo zhàng zhì dù
10	社会保障	Social security	shè huì bǎo zhàng
11	公费医疗	Healthcare with public funding	gōng fèi yī liáo
12	日本	Japan	rì běn
13	宏观管理	Macro management	hóng guān guǎn lǐ
14	医疗费	Medical fees	yī liáo fèi
15	管理	Management	guǎn lǐ
16	个人帐户	Personal account	gè rén zhàng hù
17	非处方药	Non-prescription drugs	fēi chǔ fāng yào
18	社会统筹	Overall social planning (*1)	shè huì tǒng chóu
19	医疗保健制度	Healthcare system	yī liáo bǎo jiàn zhì dù
20	市场经济	Market economy	shì chǎng jīng jì
21	健康	Health	jiàn kāng
22	研究	Research	yán jiū
23	寿命表	Life table	shòu mìng biǎo
24	经营管理	Management	jīng yíng guǎn lǐ
25	求医	Seeking doctor (accessibility to healthcare)	qiú yī
26	个人储蓄投资机制	Personal savings investment mechanism	gè rén chúxù tóuzī jīzhì
27	实践	Practice (as opposed to theories)	shí jiàn
28	制约	Restriction	zhì yuē
29	疾病基金	Sickness funds	jí bìng jī jīn
30	以药养医	Drugs to support/subsidise doctor (*2)	yǐ yào yǎng yī
31	分析	Analysis	fēn xī
32	社会保障基金	Social security fund	shè huì bǎo zhàng jī jīn
33	工资保障制度	Wage protection system	gōng zī bǎo zhàng zhì dù
34	医疗服务	Medical service	yī liáo fú wù
35	措施	Measures	cuò shī
36	基本对策	Basic countermeasure	jī běn duì cè
37	卫生部门	Health sector, health department	wèi shēng bù mén

以药养医 (yǐ yào yǎng yī) (using medicines to support/subsidise doctors/hospital management)

(1) 论"以药养医"的 内部机理 及 解决途径.

Translation: On the rationale and solution of the so-called drug-subsidising-doctors (in the Chinese medical care system) (title of the article).

(2) 本文 分析"以药养医"的 深层机理, 认为 医院 内部的 行政 主导 和 分配 制度 从根本上 造成 药价虚高, 患者 负担加重。

Translation: This paper offers an in-depth analysis of the rationale behind the so-called drug-subsidising-doctors phenomenon in China. It maintains that it is the administrative overruling and the allocation system which has caused the inflation of medical costs and the increase of burdens to the patients.

社会统筹 (shè huì tǒng chóu) (overall social planning)

(3) 从医疗保险基金筹集、收支状况、基本医疗保障、医疗费用控制、社会反映等方面, 对深圳市医疗保险新旧模式进行了比较研究, 认为社会统筹与个人帐户相结合的医疗保险新模式优于旧模式。

Translation: This paper offers a comparative analysis of the old and new models of medical insurance in the city of Shenzhen. It touches upon medical insurance pooling, balance between income and expenditure, basic medical insurance, control of medical costs, as well as the public opinion. It argues that the new medical insurance model which combines overall social planning and personal accounts is more beneficial than the old model.

(4) 如本文所分析的一样, 与中国转型时期的需要相应, 中国政府已经明确了城镇国家年金、企业年金、个人储蓄性年金"三位一体"的年金制度体系, 实行社会统筹与个人帐户相结合的多层次的模式。中国城市年金制度的筹资模式必然采用部分积累制。

Translation: As analysed in this paper, based on the practical needs from the social transition period in China, the Chinese government has stipulated a 'trinity' model for the country's pension system which encompasses state-provincial pension (governmental), corporate pension and personal saving pension. This multilevel model materialised the integration and combination of both social planning and personal accounts. The pooling model in Chinese cities will necessarily adopt the so-called partial accumulation pension system.

公费医疗 (gōng fèi yī liáo) (healthcare with public funding)

(5) 文章对已实行的三种个人医疗帐户的定义和个人帐户不够应急时的处理方法进行比较分析, 推荐"个人帐户主要用于门诊"的医疗保险模式, 并建议对于没有公费医疗和劳保医疗的社会成员只搞住院或大病保险。

Translation: This paper offered a comparison between three existing personal medical accounts and the solution to situations when personal accounts do not meet the needs in emergencies. It is in favour of the medical insurance model in which personal accounts are mainly used for regular medical consultations. It recommends hospital insurance for social members without public healthcare or labour insurance.

(6) 随着社会主义市场经济的发展和公费医疗制度改革及高等教育改革的不断深入，如何推进高校的学生医疗制度改革，建立新的安全医疗保障制度成为高校改革和发展的新课题。

Translation: A new topic that has emerged in the reform and development of Chinese universities is how to establish new secure medical insurance system to advance university student medical insurance system reform amidst the development of the socialist market economy, its public healthcare system, and the higher education reform.

医疗制度 **(yī liáo zhì dù) (healthcare system)**

(7) 我国 计划经济 时期 的 医疗保障制度 主要 集中在 公费医疗体系 的 建立、规范 和 完善 等 方面,包括 建国 初期 阶段、调整 巩固 阶段 即 规范 公费、劳保 医疗制度 阶段。

Translation: The medical security system in the planning economy period in China focused on the establishment, regulation and improvement of the public healthcare system. This includes the early period after the foundation of the PRC, and the adjustment and establishment period regarding the regulation of the public labour medical insurance system.

(8) 医疗制度改革、GMP达标、加入WTO及OTC市场竞争的加剧等，使我国制药企业的产业环境发生了巨大变化，进而对制药企业的融资策略及资本结构决策行为也构成影响。

Translation: Medicine manufacturing in China has been deeply affected by factors such as medical insurance system reform, implementation of GMP (Good Manufacturing Practice), entrance into the World Trade Organisation (WTO), as well as the escalating competition in the OTC (over-the-counter) market. These have also impacted on the financing strategies and the decision-making over capital structuring among Chinese pharmaceutical companies.

非处方药 **(fēi chǔ fāng yào) (non-prescription medicine)**

(9) 2000年1月1日起实施的我国药品分类管理制度,使得我国药品市场结构发生了巨大变化,药品市场被细分为处方药市场 (Prescription Drug Market, 简称RX市场) 和非处方药市场 (Non-prescription Drug Market, 简称OTC市场)。

Translation: The administration system of classifying medicines in China, which took effect from 1st January 2000, has led to important structural changes to the Chinese medicine market. The medicine market has been divided into Prescription Drug Market (the RX Market) and Non-Prescription Drug Market (the OTC market).

(10) 随着我国药品分类管理制度的实施,我国药品消费结构发生了变化,药品市场被细分为处方药市场 (Prescription Drug Market, 简称RX市场) 和非处方药市场 (Non-Prescription Drug Market,简称OTC市场)。

Translation: With the medication classification management system being established and implemented in China, the medicine market is divided into prescription drug market and non-prescription drug market (OTC drug market).

医院管理 (yī yuàn guǎn lǐ) (hospital management)

(11) 通过成本核算在医院管理中的应用, 总结医院开展成本核算的意义, 分析开展成本核算过程中遇到的难点, 寻找解决难点的方法, 从而更好地发挥成本分析评价和成本控制的职能, 达到降低医疗服务成本和医院运营成本的目的, 构建低成本经营优势。

Translation: Through an analysis of the implementation of cost accounting in hospital management, this paper highlights the significance of such practice in Chinese hospitals, and analyses the difficulties encountered in such a process attempting to identify practical solutions to such problems. This was to improve the functioning of cost analysis, evaluation and control, with a view to lowering the costs of medical services and hospital management to build up the market advantage.

(12) 合理用药对卫生工作现代化至关重要, 因为不合理用药加剧药害, 促成大处方泛滥, 浪费卫生资源, 损害医药人员声誉。为了盈利而开大处方导致药害加剧在近几年难以控制, 主要原因是缺乏科学的医院管理机制和信息。根治以大处方为特征的不合理用药时弊, 有必要学习"诊断相关组/预付款制度" (DRGS/PPS)。

Translation: Rational drug-use is a very important part in modern medical and health services. Irrational drug-use will aggravate drug misadventure, increase over-prescribing, waste medicinal resources and harm the reputation of medical workers. The tendency of over-prescribing for more hospital income, regardless of drug-related adverse effects, has emerged as a very serious and hard-to-control problem in recent years in China. Lack of an effective management system and necessary information may be the major causes to the problem. To systematically change such a situation, it is necessary to study Diagnosis-related group (DRG) and Medicare Prospective Payment Systems (PPS).

医疗保险制度 (yī liáo bǎo xiǎn zhì dù) (medical insurance system)

(13) 镇江自1995年初试行医疗保险制度以来,试点医院的运行出现了一些新的机制特征,面临着一组新的经济矛盾,主要是制度变迁、宏观经济环境、历史存量、微观管理滞后以及对医院的性质、地位和作用缺乏合理的认识等因素导致。解决新问题的关键在于:一是合理界定医院的性质、地位和作用,二是确定新的"三位一体"的改革思路,三是运用系统论的整体观、目的观、相关观制定医院发展策略。

Translation: Since medical insurance was first introduced in the village of Zhenjiang in early 1995, a new set of systematic problems and economic conflicts has emerged in hospitals piloting the new medical insurance. These have been caused by the transition of the medical insurance system, macro-economic environment, historical problems, ineffective micro-administration and lack of understanding of the role and function of hospitals. The key to solving these problems consists in firstly, a reasonable definition of the role and function of hospitals; secondly, establishment of the new so-called 'trinity' reform; and thirdly, development of growth strategies for hospitals using the principles of system theories, i.e. integration, purposefulness and relevance.

(14) 论述了面对医疗服务的供需变化应采取的基本对策: 推行区域卫生规划, 实现卫生资源优化配置; 实现医疗管理体制整体化, 医疗系统管理行业化, 坚持医院分级管理和医院评审, 调整和健全医疗服务体系; 推进医疗保险制度的实施, 促使卫生资源的合理调整: 利用经济手段疏导需求, 引导资源的配置流向; 强化资源立法。

Translation: This study discusses some basic countermeasures that should be adopted for the changing demand and supply of medical services which include promotion of regional health planning; implementation of optimised health resources allocation; integration of health administration; professionalisation of health system management; adherence to tiered hospital management and assessment; adjustment and improvement of medical services; advancement of health insurance system; rational adjustment of health resources allocation which requires the use of economic means to moderate demands and supplies in order to direct the allocation of resources; and the strengthening of resources legislation.

The list of keywords identified in the CNKI database (see Table 3.1) were the top frequency content words or multiword expressions related to the search word 'healthcare insurance system'. These keywords provide useful information regarding the strategic focuses, priorities and particular approaches to the problems encountered in the structural change and reform of the healthcare and social security system in China up to the end of the 1990s. Some of the words, especially multiword expressions, are heavily culturally loaded expressions which were formed or created through lexical variations of existing Chinese fixed or idiomatic expressions.

In order to understand contrasts and differences between the Chinese context and global healthcare research prioritisation and agenda setting represented by the WHO 2000 Annual Report, a list of keywords in the WHO 2000 report which focus on the development of more robust health insurance to tackle growing health financial risks in developing countries including China is shown in Table 3.2. The extraction of keywords from the WHO 2000 Report was different from the extraction of keywords from Chinese publications collected in the CNKI database. Keywords in Table 3.2 were identified by comparing the full text of the WHO 2000 Annual Report with a large collection of WHO annual reports published between 1990 and 2013. The large corpus of the WHO reports between 1990 and 2013 served as the reference corpus in the cross-corpus comparison. This statistical comparison method is widely used in corpus linguistics (Anthony 2013; Hunt and Harvey 2015). The statistical method used was log-likelihood.

The two keyword-lists (Table 3.1 for China; Table 3.2 for the WHO) exhibit associated yet distinct lexical patterns of medical terminologies which belong to and reflect two analytical and research systems operating at national and international levels. For example, the top frequency word 'system' in Table 3.2 (WHO health policy terminology in English) has strong connection with similar keywords shown in Table 3.1 (Chinese health policy terminology), in which the English keyword 'system' was linked with more specific, socially and culturally contextualised Chinese multiword expressions such as 'medical insurance system' (yī liáo bǎo xiǎn zhì dù), 'social security system' (shè huì bǎo zhàng zhì dù), 'health care system' (yī liáo bǎo jiàn zhì dù), 'wage protection system' (gōng zī bǎo zhàng zhì dù).

Keywords in Table 3.2 (English health terminology) such as 'distribution' and 'regulation' are related to keywords in Table 3.1 (Chinese health policy terminology) such as 'total volume control' (zǒng liàng kòng zhì); 'overall social planning' (shè huì tǒng chóu), 'structural adjustment' (jié gòu tiáo zhěng) and even Chinese health-domain-specific idiomatic expressions like the controversial practice of 'using over-prescription to support or to subsidise doctors' (yǐ yào yǎng yī) which describe and highlight practical problems and social issues specific to national health policies developed and experimented in the Chinese culture and society when its

Table 3.2   List of keywords in the WHO 2000 Annual Report

No.	Frequency	Keyness[a]	Keywords in the WHO 2000 Annual Report
1	480	342.777	System
2	126	196.422	Stewardship
3	261	196.38	Private
4	193	176.068	Providers
5	108	171.532	Responsiveness
7	123	133.454	Incentives
8	185	127.869	Performance
11	69	109.915	Fairness
12	97	107.202	Pooling
16	77	98.619	Capital
19	78	90.545	Market
21	75	85.411	Purchasing
23	134	81.221	Insurance
24	69	78.821	Contribution
26	98	68.785	Distribution
27	42	67.259	Rank
28	64	66.933	Provider
32	165	65.499	Financing
38	36	58.7	Equality
39	55	58.164	Prepayment
40	175	56.309	Poor
43	42	49.816	Consumers
44	79	49.701	Disability
45	59	49.122	Index
46	54	48.796	Regulation
47	320	48.618	Child
48	56	46.811	Functions
49	140	46.086	Financial
50	25	44.657	Hierarchical
51	39	44.051	Achievement
52	51	43.71	Adjusted
53	31	43.456	Competition
54	53	43.189	Relative
56	55	42.355	Finance
57	48	42.327	Physicians
58	29	42.15	Recurrent
59	36	41.981	Rules
60	25	41.654	Rationing
61	42	41.212	Objectives

[a]Word keyness was computed using log-likelihood method

primary healthcare system underwent important transition and structural reforms.

In order to establish effective communication between international health policy-making and national audiences, it is essential to develop well-structured bi-directional (i.e. translation in two directions) bilingual health policy terminologies which incorporate both international and national (or language- and culture-specific) terms. This bi-directional or multidirectional health policy translation is currently lacking in many authoritative international health agencies, whereby the vast majority of official documents are selected and translated from English into the target languages. This has overlooked the importance and critical needs to inform audiences of inherent differences between international and national health policy-making, further hampering the exchange and growth of specialised knowledge in different social and cultural systems.

With the availability of large-scale digital resources and corpus mining tools and techniques, it is now feasible to identify keywords in national research and official publications such as CHKI database. The automatic identification and extraction of such keywords make important preparation for the development of much-needed bi-directional terminologies in English and the target languages for specialised professional translation. This is a largely underexplored research area which holds the key to the effective cross-cultural and cross-lingual communication of health policy issues, as well as the construction of much-needed consensus and cooperation to tackle pressing health problems between international health organisations, national stakeholders and the general public.

References

Anthony, L. 2013. A Critical Look at Software Tools in Corpus Linguistics. *Linguistic Research* 30 (2): 141–161.

Barber, S.L., M. Borowitz, H. Bekedam, and J. Ma. 2013. The Hospital of the Future in China: China's Reform of Public Hospitals and Trends from Industrialized Countries. *Health Policy and Planning.* doi:10.1093/heapol/czt023.

Fang, G., J. Lu, and M. Shi. 2015. Analysis of the Origin of Drug to Support Doctor and Countermeasures. *China Hospital Management* 35 (7): 5–6.

Hua, H.H.Z.J.W., and C.M.Z. Su. 2003. Comparison and Study on Online Chinese Periodical Full-Text Databases of CNKI and VIP. *New Technology of Library and Information Service* 6: 18.

Hunt, D., and K. Harvey. 2015. Health Communication and Corpus Linguistics: Using Corpus Tools to Analyse Eating Disorder Discourse Online. In *Corpora and Discourse Studies*, 134–154. London: Palgrave Macmillan.

Li, L.I.U. 2007. Further Exploitation and Utilization of the Retrieval Function of CNKI. *Journal of Academic Library and Information Science* 1: 014.

Li, J., Z. Liu, R. Chen, D. Hu, W. Li, X. Li, X. Chen, B. Huang, and L. Liao. 2014. The Quality of Reports of Randomized Clinical Trials on Traditional Chinese Medicine Treatments: A Systematic Review of Articles Indexed in the China National Knowledge Infrastructure database from 2005 to 2012. *BMC Complementary and Alternative Medicine* 14 (1): 1.

Lin, Yuhong. 2013. The Reform and Development about the Distribution System of Profits of State-Owned Enterprises. *Business and Globalization* 1: 35–39.

Liu, X.B. 2013. Bibliometric Analysis of the Republic of China Literature Based on CNKI Database. *New Century Library* 8: 008.

Shen, J.J., S. Zhou, L. Xu, J. Chen, C.R. Cochran, and E.R. Fisher. 2014. Effects of the New Health Care Reform on Hospital Performance in China: A Seven-Year Trend from 2005 to 2011. *Journal of Health Care Finance* 41 (1).

Wang, G., and L. Wang. 2015. Analysis on the Results of Agricultural Science and Technology Literature Retrieval based on CNKI, Wanfang and VIP Retrieval Platform. *Agriculture Network Information* 7: 016.

World Health Organisation 2000 Annual Report. *Health Systems: Improving Performance*. Available at http://www.who.int/whr/2000/en/whr00_en.pdf.

CHAPTER 4

Construction of an English-Chinese Parallel Corpus of WHO Health Translation

Abstract This chapter introduces the construction of a parallel English-Chinese corpus of WHO health translations. It gives details of the practical consideration in the collection of corpus materials to build the parallel corpus. The construction of the parallel corpus facilitates the identification and extraction of English health risk terms which gave rise to competing translations or the detected terminological variation in health translation, the translation phenomenon highlighted in this chapter and discussed at length in this book. The variant translations extracted in the parallel corpus exploration were grouped into different clusters of health risk terminologies that underscored the development and building of new health risks knowledge among the target audiences.

Keywords Parallel corpus construction · Health financial risk Terminology variation

4.1 Practical Considerations in the Parallel Corpus Construction

Specialised translation such as health translation entails both advanced translation skills between two languages and a thorough, in-depth understanding of the key topics and research methodologies discussed in the source text materials. To produce high-quality and accessible specialised translation such as health policy guidelines, first and foremost, it is

© The Author(s) 2017   31
M. Ji, *Translation and Health Risk Knowledge Building in China*,
DOI 10.1007/978-981-10-4681-0_4

essential to develop via close collaboration between domain specialists and translators, cross-lingual terminologies to be deployed consistently throughout the entire translation workflow. Terminological inconsistency which may well occur in the absence of coordinated specialised translation can lead to substantial confusion in the dissemination of original source materials and complicate the development of national health resources in line with international health policy guidelines.

A main research focus in empirical translation studies is the evaluation and assessment of the lexical consistency of translation terminologies. Aligned parallel corpora between the source and the target texts have been introduced to corpus-based translation studies since the early 2000s (Laviosa 2002; Olohan 2004). These purposely designed digital translation resources can effectively enable the systematic search and empirical contrastive analysis of translated terms. For the purpose of this study, parallel corpora were constructed with carefully selected bilingual texts. Three main considerations were behind this choice of original English health materials. Firstly, while WHO produces on a yearly basis global health reports drawing upon latest public health research, the 2000 Report was directly related to health financial risks as the main focus of the present study.

Secondly, the availability of full-text instead of segment-based Chinese translation of WHO health policy materials was also an important factor, as this may well impact the corpus-based comparative analysis between English source texts and the Chinese translations. Large translation projects often require substantial intellectual input and cross-institute and trans-disciplinary cooperation. Large translation projects are often labour-intensive and expensive to deliver, especially when end products are of importance for international and national policy-making, for example, the translation of the WHO health reports.

To solve this practical issue of producing high-quality translations taking into account substantial costs involved, a normal practice at international organisations like the WHO is to select a number of official publications of global or regional importance; and organise in-house translators to work on the materials; or to outsource the translation of selected materials to reputable national research institutes, accredited translation agencies, or not-for-profit organisations in different locations around the world.

It is well known that apart from English, there are five official WHO working languages, i.e. Arabic, Chinese, French, Spanish and Russian. Often, the policy documents and materials developed by the WHO and chosen for translation into other languages reflect the relevance and importance of the research for the countries and communities with particular language, cultural and social backgrounds. Abridged and edited translations present another practical and effective approach to disseminate WHO health research findings to a global audience in a timely and efficient manner.

In the current study, full-text translation was preferred, as it can afford sufficient corpus data for the extraction and analysis of the use of distinct linguistic expressions as variant translations. This is essential for this study which focuses on the comparative analysis of variant translations and their differing uses in naturally occurring texts in the target language. However, for practical reasons, when compared to extensive WHO materials in English, a limited number of strategic policy documents have full-text translations into the other five official languages of the organisation.

The WHO Annual Report, *Health Systems: Improving Performance* (Geneva, Switzerland 2000a), is one of the few English policy documents which have been translated in full into simplified Chinese, the common language used in mainland China. This is also the language of the large-scale Chinese scientific and media databases used in this study, for example, the CNKI database (for details see Chap. 5) for the original Chinese linguistic analysis.

Thirdly, in order to analyse patterns of the academic and media dissemination of health expressions related to health risk concepts, the production date of the translation of international health policy documents should allow the collection of longitudinal publication data in sufficient quantities. This is especially important for the current study which aims to develop statistical indicators to measure the social impact or the media uptake of specialised health translation materials developed for national audiences. The WHO 2000 Annual Report and its simplified Chinese version proved the most suitable source and target textual materials to address the key research aims and goals of the present study.

4.2   VARIATION IN THE TRANSLATION OF HEALTH RISK TERMINOLOGIES

As described in the previous section, the textual analysis started with the corpus-driven identification and retrieval of conceptual clusters of health financial risk terms. Conceptual clusters contain a variety of linguistic expressions or *synonyms* that may well serve as variant translations in the target language. It should be noted that the definition of 'synonym' in this study differs from the dictionary meaning. In original and natural languages—as opposed to translated languages, for example, English or Chinese—synonyms are words which may largely replace each other in the textual context given their semantic similarity. This study focuses on the selective use of linguistic expressions in the target language for translation purposes. As a result, a group of words are extracted, highlighted and labelled as *synonyms* when they tend to be used to translate particular source language words.

These 'translation synonyms' are identified based on their association with source text expressions, in terms of their cross-lingual matching patterns revealed in the translational corpus analysis, instead of their semantic similarity or proximity to each other in the target language. For example, the corpus analysis of the WHO health policy translation shows that Chinese words and expressions meaning 'dangerous element', 'dangerous factor' and 'risk factor' are constantly deployed interchangeably by the translators to interpret the original English expression *risk factor*. These linguistic expressions are certainly not seen as synonyms in the Chinese language but they are extracted and grouped under the conceptual cluster 'risk factor' (fēng xiǎn yīn sù) in the current study, as they have proven to be conceptually linked variant translations in the parallel corpus which has been constructed for the study of Chinese translations of the WHO policy guidelines for global health risk prevention and management mechanisms, especially in the developing world.

A parallel corpus of the WHO 2000 Annual Report and its full-text Chinese translation was first constructed (WHO 2000b Annual Report, simplified Chinese version: *She Jie Wei Sheng Bao Gao: Wei Sheng Xi Tong, Gai Jin Ye Ji,* Beijing). The parallel corpus contained sentence-by-sentence alignment between the source and the target texts. The sentence-level alignment was a laborious and extremely time-consuming but highly rewarding process (Teich 2003; Chen and Ng 1989; Al-Amer et al. 2015). In the process of bilingual text alignment, interesting and revealing cross-lingual matching patterns began to emerge. It was found that a number of Chinese translations of English health financial risk terms exhibited varying levels of semantic variation and alteration of the original English expressions (see Table 4.1).

After the construction of the parallel English-Chinese corpus, a full-text search of the word 'risk' was conducted in the original WHO 2000 English report. This initial search extracted a very large number of risk-related expressions and terms. However, not all of these terms were relevant for the analysis of health translation, particularly for the study of variant translations in the current study, which represent different cross-lingual lexical experiments motivated by different translation strategies. The focus of the manual screening process following the automatic search was therefore put on the retrieval of English health financial risk expressions which had given rise to a variety of translation options seen as variant translations in this study. Such linguistic variations point to a shared underlying conceptual cluster of health risks highlighted for investigation in this study. The detection and retrieval of such conceptual clusters of health financial risks require an in-depth contrastive linguistic analysis of both the original English source text and its Mandarin Chinese translations.

In the manual screening process, one went through a very large number of sentence pairs in English and Chinese to identify variant translations, instances of mistranslations were discarded or marked with an asterisk * in the corpus annotation, as they were not seen as relevant for this study that has a focus on context- or strategy-motivated translation variation, instead of translation quality assessment. In order to develop new empirical analytical approaches to the study of specialised translation, this study investigates the widely existent phenomenon of variant translations in health translation.

It is believed that the selective use of translation methods and techniques underscores the mediated *interaction* between two distinct linguistic, cultural and knowledge systems which are on the one hand, the international health knowledge system and on the other hand, the Chinese health knowledge system which was developing rapidly since the mid-twentieth century. Translation has long played an instrumental role in disseminating scientific knowledge and bridging the gap between cultures and societies. This is fully illustrated in this study which offers an empirical analysis of the development of health financial risk concepts and terms in modern Chinese in the late 1990s.

Table 4.1 Summary of Chinese variant translations of WHO health financial risk terms

No.	English expression	Chinese variant translation
Fixed expressions		
219	At a high [**risk**] of	有着 高 [风险] (risk)
65*	At greater than usual [**risk**] of ill-health	比 通常的疾病 与 健康 [危险] 比率 都 高 (danger)
263	At [**risk**] of impoverishment	有 贫困 [危险] (danger)
55	At [**risk**] of impoverishment	处于 贫困的[危险]中 (danger)
89*	On the basis of [**risk**]	[危险]基线的程度 (danger)
51	*Ex ante* [**risk**]	事先[风险] (risk)
Financial risk		
225	Financial [**risk**]	财政 [风险] (risk)
125	Financial [**risk**]	融资 [风险] (risk)
113	Financial [**risk**]	财政 [风险] (risk)
107	Financial [**risk**]	财务 [风险] (risk)
93	Financial [**risk**]	财政 [危险] (danger)
91	Financial [**risk**]	财政 [风险] (risk)
87	Financial [**risk**]	财政 [危险] (danger)
63	Financial [**risk**]	财政 [危险] (danger)
27	Financial [**risk**]	资金 [风险] (risk)
25	Financial [**risk**]	财务 [风险] (risk)
23	Financial [**risk**]	财政 [风险] (risk)
15	Financial [**risk**]	财政 [风险] (risk)
9	Financial [**risk**]	财政 [风险] (risk)
129	Financial [**risk**]	出资 [风险] (risk)
261	Financial [**risk**]	资助 [风险] (risk)
191	Financial [**risk**]	财政 [风险] (risk)
111	Financial [**risk**]	[风险] (risk)
101	Financial [**risk**]	投资 [风险] (risk)
43	Financial [**risk**]	金融 [风险] (risk)
Risk factor		
253	[**Risk factors**]	[危险因素] (dangerous factor)
81	[**Risk factors**]	[危险因子] (dangerous element)
77	[**Risk factors**]	[危险因子] (dangerous element)
73	[**Risk factors**]	[危险因子] (dangerous element)
71	[**Risk factors**]	[危险因子] (dangerous element)
69	[**Risk factors**]	[危险因子] (dangerous element)
13	[**Risk factors**]	[风险因素] (dangerous factor)
11	[**Risk factors**]	[危险因素] (dangerous factor)
83	[**Risk factors**]	[危险因子] (dangerous element)
79	Patterns of [**risk**]	[危险因子] 形式 (dangerous element)

(continued)

Table 4.1 (continued)

No.	English expression	Chinese variant translation
75*	Preventable [**risk factors**]	预防性 [危险因子] (dangerous element)
59*	Common [**risk factor**]	普遍的[危险因子] (dangerous element)
45	Health [**risk**]	健康 [风险] (risk)
Types of risks		
39	[**Risk**] of coverage being denied	拒保的[危险] (danger)
185	[**Risk**] of fragmenting the pool	集资分散的[风险] (risk)
103	[**Risk**] of having to pay	付费的[风险] (risk)
41	[**Risk**] of illness	疾病的[危险] (danger)
37	Substantial [**risk**]	实质性的[风险] (risk)
259	Underlying [**risks**] of death	潜在死亡[风险] (risk)
Risk-derived concepts		
117	[**Risk**]-based contribution systems	基于[风险] 的出资系统 (risk)
21	[**Risk**]-based insurance schemes	以 [风险] 为基础的保险制度 (risk)
257	[**Risk**]-based schemes	[风险] 基础上的方案 (risk)
193	[**Risk**]-related	[风险] 相关 (risk)
211	[**Risk**]-related contributions	[风险] 相关的出资 (risk)
135	[**Risk**]-related cross-subsidies	[风险] 相关的交叉资助 (risk)
197	[**Risk**]-related health insurance	[风险] 相关的卫生保险 (risk)
51	[**Risk**]-related insurance premium	与 [风险] 有关的保险费 (risk)
49	[**Risk**]-related payments	[风险性] 支付 (risky)
47	[**Risk**] associated with out-of-pocket payments	与现金支付有关的 [风险] (risk)
161	Non-[**risk**]-related contribution	非[风险]相关的 出资 (risk)
159	Non-[**risk**]-related contribution	非[风险]相关的 出资 (risk)
197	Non-[**risk**]-related contribution	非[风险]相关的出资 (risk)
167	Non-[**risk**]-related contributions	非[风险]相关的出资 (risk)
Risk categorisation		
201	[**Risk**] category	[风险]级别 (risk)
199	[**Risk**] category	[风险]级别 (risk)
61	High [**risk**] pregnancies	高[危]妊娠 (danger)
237	High-[**risk**] members	高[风险]会员 (risk)
203	High-[**risk**] members	高[风险]的成员 (risk)
217	Highest [**risk**] group	最高[风险因素]人群 (risk factor)
249	Lower-[**risk**] groups	低[风险]人群 (risk)
Risk compensation and cross-subsidisation		
221	[**Risk**] compensation mechanisms	[风险]补偿机制 (risk)
169	[**Risk**] compensation mechanisms	[风险]补偿机制 (risk)
137	[**Risk**] cross-subsidisation	[风险]相关的交叉资助 (risk)

(continued)

Table 4.1 (continued)

No.	English expression	Chinese variant translation
101	Cross-subsidies from low to high health [**risk**]	低健康 [危险因素] (dangerous factors) 到 高健康 [危险因素] (dangerous factors) 交叉资助
131	Coss-subsidies from low to high [**risk**]	由 低[风险] (risk) 朝向 高[风险] (risk) 交叉资助
127*	Cross-subsidies from low-[**risk**] to high-[**risk**] individual	由 高[风险] (risk) 人群 向 低[风险] (risk) 人群 进行的交叉资助
Risk equalisation		
205	Risk [**equalisation**]	风险[公平化] (equalisation)
139*	Risk [**equalisation**]	风险 [公平性 机制] (fairness mechanism)
153*	Central risk [**equalisation**] fund	集中风险 [公平性] 基金 (fairness)
Risk handling strategies—spreading risks		
133	[Spread risk]	分散投资风险 (spread investment risks)
119	[Spread risk]	分散风险 (spread risks)
155	[Spreading of risk]	分散投资风险 (spread investment risks)
147	[Spreading of risk]	分散投资风险 (spread investment risks)
183	[Spreading risk]	风险分担 (risk sharing)
151	[Spreading risk]	风险分散 (risk spreading)
3	[Spreading risk]	分散投资风险 (spread investment risks)
1	[Spreading risk]	分散投资风险 (spread investment risks)
109	Degree of [spreading of risk]	风险分散程度 (risk-spreading level)
149	[Redistribute risk]	分散风险 (spread risks)
5	[Redistribute risk]	分散风险 (spread risks)
Risk handling strategies—risk pooling		
245	[Risk pool]	风险共保集团 (risk commonly-insured group)
251	[Risk pooling]	风险共保 (risk commonly-insured)
243	[Risk pooling]	风险共保 (risk commonly-insured)
239	[Risk pooling]	风险共保 (risk commonly-insured)
235	[Risk pooling]	风险共担 (risk commonly-insured)
231	[Risk pooling]	风险共保 (risk commonly-insured)
19	[Risk pooling]	风险集资 (risk financing)
17	[Risk pooling]	风险集资 (risk financing)
7	[Risk pooling]	风险共担 (risk commonly-insured)

Table 4.1 (continued)

No.	English expression	Chinese variant translation
255	[Risk pools]	风险共保集团 (risk commonly-insured group)
Risk handling strategies—risk selection		
233	[Risk selection]	风险选择 (risk selection)
231	[Risk selection]	风险选择 (risk selection)
229	[Risk selection]	风险选择 (risk selection)
223	[Risk selection]	风险选择 (risk selection)
215	[Risk selection]	风险选择 (risk selection)
165	[Risk selection]	风险选择 (risk selection)
85	[Risk selection]	危险选择 (danger selection)
213	[Risk-selected]	依照低风险原则 (based on low-risk principles)
Risk handling strategies—risk sharing		
175	[Risk sharing]	风险分担 (risk sharing)
179	[Risk sharing] agreement	风险分担协议 (risk sharing)
177	[Risk sharing] payment mechanism	风险分担支付机制 (risk sharing)
187	[Risk sharing] payment mechanisms	风险分担型的支付机制 (risk-sharing-model)
183	[Risk sharing] payment mechanisms	风险分担的支付机制 (risk sharing)
57	[Risk sharing] schemes	风险承担方案 (risk-bearing)
173	[Risk sharing]	风险承担 (risk-bearing)
181	[Risk sharing]	风险分担 (risk-sharing)
34	[Risk sharing]	风险分担 (risk-sharing)
Risk handling strategies—risk capitation		
247	[Risk-adjusted] per capital payments	人均风险调整付款 (average risk adjustment payment)
171	[Risk-adjusted] capitation	风险调整的人头税 (risk adjustment tax per head)
209	Risk adjustment	风险调节 (risk adjustment)
157	Adjusting for the average risk of a group	根据某一人群的平均危险因素作出调节 (adjustment based on average dangerous factors of a population group)
195	[Non-risk-adjusted] capitation payment	非风险调整人头税支付 (non-risk-adjustment tax per head payment)

Number on the left column indicates the aligned sentence sequence in Appendix

In the parallel corpus analysis, English source expressions were extracted from the large search result list when it was found that the conceptual complexity of English health policy terms was reflected in the emergence of a number of variant translations in the Chinese version of the 2000 WHO annual report. Variant translations were then identified in the Chinese part of the parallel corpus and grouped into conceptual clusters labelled with the original English text expressions. That is to say, these conceptually linked Chinese linguistic expressions or *variant translations,* as defined and highlighted in this corpus-based translation analysis, were found based on their observed links or co-occurrence patterns with a shared English source term in the parallel English and Chinese translation database.

Once extracted from the parallel English-Chinese corpus, these variant translations were analysed with large-scale original Chinese research and media databases, i.e. the CNKI database, in an effort to identify subtle differences in their semantic meaning and their distinct use in specific domains and research disciplines in the target language, i.e. Mandarin Chinese, the common language in mainland China. This helps to yield further insights into the translation process through which health translators experiment with different translation options and strategies by creating variant translations of original English health policy materials in the largely developing Chinese public health knowledge system.

The comparison among translated health terms in the target language reveals different translation tactics and strategies used by translators working on the same English source document. This requires a close observation of the distribution and use of these variant translations within the Chinese cultural and language context. The next section presents some examples of these translation variations, which although are not necessarily synonyms in original Chinese, they have been used as variant translations as shown in the parallel corpus analysis. They were manually extracted from more than 500 health risk-related bilingual term pairs collected in the aligned English-Chinese corpus of the 2000 WHO annual report, as they illustrate how the interpretation of the English source text by translators may well impact on the understanding and perception of the importance, urgency and relevance of the original materials among the target audience.

Examples of Chinese Variant Translations of the 2000 WHO Annual Report
The search word used for systematically analysing the English source text is 'risk'.

English Source Text (ST)
The 2000a *World Health Organisation Report: Health Systems: Improving Performance,* World Health Organisation, Geneva, Switzerland

Chinese Translation Text (TT)
世界卫生报告：卫生系统, 改进业绩
    (shì jiè wèi shēng bào gào: wèi shēng xì tǒng, gǎi jìn yè jī)
(November 2000)
    Translated and published by Chinese People's Health Press, Beijing
    Table 4.1 gives a systematic review of the translation of risk-related terms and expressions in the original WHO English health report. As we can see, lexical translation variation exists widely across a range of risk terms and expressions which lie at the heart of the WHO global health report. Different types of lexical variation which reflect distinct translation strategies deployed when the WHO document was first translated into Chinese were identified based on the systematic bilingual corpus analysis: firstly, the use of conceptually associated yet distinct nouns, for example, using 'danger', 'dangerous factor' or 'risky factor' to translate 'risk' and 'risk factor'.
    Secondly, the replacement of nouns indicating actions and procedures with nouns indicating qualities of systems or entities, for example, translating 'equalisation' which was an important item in the WHO health policy guidelines with 'fairness' of the healthcare system. A similar case was echoed in the translation of '(risk-adjusted) capitation' with an existing Chinese idiom *rén tóu shuì* or poll or head tax which was borrowed from classical Chinese to refer to a traditional taxation practice that had existed in the feudal Chinese societies from as early as the Qin Dynasty (221 BC–207 BC) (Du 2008). The corpus analysis revealed that that the semantic meaning of such important items in the WHO health policy guidelines was heavily socially contextualised and culturally reinterpreted in the cross-lingual translation process. This translation strategy, on the one hand, greatly facilitated the understanding by the target audience, and on the other hand, reduced the intended effect and function of the

global health policy document to promote social reforms within the Chinese cultural and health knowledge context.

Thirdly, lexical variation showed to be evident mostly in the translation of new health policy concepts which did not exist in the Chinese health policy vocabulary—typical examples were terms clustered under 'risk pooling' and 'risk adjustment'. The unnatural and sometimes rather awkward lexico-syntactic structure of the translations provided implies confusion among translators working at the time regarding the interpretation of the semantic meaning of the original English terms and expressions, as well as the creation and establishment of appropriate translations in the target language of Chinese.

Although far from being an exhaustive list of the translation strategies for interpreting health policy materials, these three sets of identified translation methods, which were identified through the corpus-based analysis of a large number of lexical variations in the Chinese version of the WHO policy document, have provided us with useful insights into issues and problems in health policy translation. It seems to suggest that in translating health policy materials, a **balanced** translation model which takes into account both the reading habits of the target audience, for example, using culturally and linguistically conventionalised lexical constructs and widely accepted expressions, and the strategic foregrounding of important scientific knowledge in the international health policy guidelines, for instance, through the creation of new translated terms to highlight suggested courses of action and approaches to social and healthcare reforms by international health agencies like 'risk pooling' and 'risk equalisation' are most desirable and effective. The aligned textual excerpts given below provide more details of the textual context in which variant health translations were identified in the corpus-based contrastive linguistic analysis.

CONCEPTUAL CLUSTER: RISK FACTOR

1. To make matters more complicated, a given intervention may be effective against more than one disease or cause, because it works on a common ***risk factor*** or symptom.

   Chinese translation: 使 问题 更加 复杂化 的 是,某一 特定 的 干预 会 作用 于 一个 以上 的 疾病 或 病因, 因为 其 作用 于 一个 普遍的 <u>危险因子</u> (wéi xiǎn yīn zǐ) *(dangerous element)* 或 症状。

2. Major progresses have been made recently in understanding global health and disease patterns, including analysis of ***risk factors*** which influence several diseases at once.

   Chinese translation: 最近, 人们 已经 在 了解 全球 卫生 和 疾病 形式 方面 获得 了 很大 的 进展, 这 包括 对 能够 立即 影响 严重 疾病 <u>危险因子</u> (wéi xiǎn yīn zǐ) (*dangerous elements*) 的 分析.

3. The public health services in a given country should attempt to deal with such preventable ***risk factors***, taking account of local contexts.

   Chinese translation: 某一 确定 国家的 公共 卫生 服务 应该 力图 解决 这些 预防性 <u>危险因子</u> (wéi xiǎn yīn zǐ) *(dangerous elements)*, 也 包括 当地的 各种 因素.

4. Introducing regulations such as community rating (adjusting for the average ***risk*** of a group), portable employment-based pooling (insurance that a worker keeps when changing jobs)...may pave the way for larger pooling in the future.

   Chinese translation: 引入 各种 调节 机制, 如 社区 评估(根据 某一 人群的 平均 <u>危险 因素</u> (wéi xiǎn yīn sù) *(danger factors)* 作出 调节)、可携带的 基于 工作的 集资(当 工作者 更换工作 时 可以 继续 保持的 保险)··· 就可以 在 为 集资体的 参与者 提供 保障的 同时 为 未来的 大型化的 集资 铺平 道路。

5. Local and national ***risk factors*** need to be understood.

   Chinese translation: 需要 了解 地方的 和 全国的 <u>危险因素</u> (wéi xiǎn yīn sù) *(dangerous factors)*.

6. Other major ***risk factors*** include unsafe sex, alcohol, indoor pollution, tobacco...and hypertension.

   Chinese translation: 其他 主要 <u>危险 因子</u> (wéi xiǎn yīn zǐ) *(dangerous elements)* 包括 不安全的 性 活动、酒精, 室内 污染、烟草、... 高血压.

7. Fair financing in health systems means that the ***risks*** each household faces due to the costs of the health system are distributed according to ability to pay rather than to ***the risk of illness***.

   Chinese translation: 卫生系统 的 合理 的 融资 是指, 根据 支付 能力 而非 <u>疾病 的 危险</u> (jí bìng de wéi xiǎn) *(the dangers of diseases)* 来 分散 每个 家庭 因 支付 卫生系统 的 花费 而 面临的 <u>风险</u> (fēng xiǎn) *(risks)*.

These aligned textual excerpts were identified and extracted automatically by using 'risk' as the search word in the exploration of the English-Chinese parallel corpus constructed for this study. As may be seen from the cross-lingual analysis, the word 'risk' and its high-frequency collocation 'risk factor' were translated in at least three different ways which were 'dangerous elements' (wéi xiǎn yīn zǐ), 'dangerous factors' (wéi xiǎn yīn sù) and the more recent health policy concept 'risk' (fēng xiǎn). The lexical and semantic differences among these translation variations may not be as significant for non-specialised audiences as for specialised readers. However, such differences may cause distinct ways to interpret the original source text, especially when the use and distribution of these translation variations does not seem to show consistent patterns across the translated document.

Now let us take a close look at the layers of semantic differences among the translation variations found. First, the Chinese word *wéi xiǎn* (danger) is distinctly different from the expression *fēng xiǎn* (risk). While the former indicates clearly defined harms, the latter which was a very new concept in health policy-making in the 1990s in China refers to external and/or internal conditions that may potentially or likely to cause negative impact on the subject or object under study. The corpus analysis clearly shows that the Chinese translators used the word *wéi xiǎn* (danger) much more frequently than the more accurate yet less familiar translation *fēng xiǎn* (risk) in the translation of the WHO original document.

Second, it was found in the translational corpus analysis that in dealing with high-frequency word collocations such as 'risk factor', two lexical variations co-exist throughout the Chinese translation: 危险 因 子 (wéi xiǎn yīn zǐ) *(dangerous elements)* and 危险因素 (wéi xiǎn yīn sù) *(dangerous factors)*. At first sight, the two Chinese translations seem to be similar to each other, but if the translation resources were developed for professional use such as for health policy-makers and academic research, it is necessary to delineate and highlight the important semantic differences between the two Chinese words yīn zǐ (*elements*) and yīn sù (*factors*). For native Chinese speakers, the word *yīn zǐ* tends to be more frequently used for internal conditions or components of a system or an object, as the monosyllabic word *zǐ* literally mean 'something little, offspring or a small part'. On the other hand, the word *yīn sù* tends to be used to refer to external conditions and factors that may affect the subject. In both cases, the initial monosyllabic word *yīn* indicates a causal or contributing relationship.

It became clear in the parallel corpus analysis that the Chinese translators had been using these two words indiscriminately to translate the original English expression 'risk factor', although the Chinese word *yīn zǐ* may be better used to refer to describe and analyse diseases; the Chinese word *yīn sù* should have been used consistently and systematically for the purpose of social and policy analyses. It was revealing to notice that the translators used two different words *wēi xiǎn* (danger) and the word *fēng xiǎn* (risk) to translate the English expression 'risk' in the same sentence (No. 7) which points to a lack of consistent and verified bilingual terminology for health policy translation at the time.

CONCEPTUAL CLUSTER: EQUALISATION

1. Pooling by itself allows for ***equalisation of contributions*** among members of the pool regardless of their financial risk associated with service utilisation. It also allows the low-risk poor to subsidise the high-risk rich.
   Chinese translation: 集资 本身 容许 在 不考虑 每个 参与者 使用 卫生 服务 的 出资 风险 的 前提下, 将 出资 份额 平均 分摊 *(equal sharing of financial contributions)* 到 集资 参与者 的 每个人 头上, 而且 其 也 容许 低风险 的 穷人 去 资助 高风险 的 富人。

2. Cross-subsidisation can also occur among members of different pools (in a multiple pool system) via explicit ***risk and income equalisation***, such as those being used in the social security systems of Argentina, Colombia and the Netherlands.
   Chinese translation: 对于 含 多个 集资体 的 系统,交叉 资助 也 可 以 通过 明确的 风险 公平性 及 收入 公平性 机制 *(fairness of risks and fair mechanisms of incomes)* 出现于 不同 集资体 中 的 集资 参 与者 之间, 如 阿根廷、哥伦比亚、荷兰 等 国家 所实行的 就是 这样的 机制。

3. Even under single pool organisations, decentralisation, unless accompanied by ***equalisation for resource allocation***, may result in significant risk and income differences among decentralised regions.
   Chinese translation: 即使 是 单一的 集资组织, 除非 伴有 公平的 资 源 分配 机制 *(a fair mechanism for resource allocation)*, 否则 分散化 可能 在 分散的 区域 之间 导致 显著的 风险 和 收入 的 差异。

4. Some health systems with multiple social security organisations have introduced central collecting agencies in charge of ***risk***

**equalisation** among pools (as in Colombia, Germany and the Netherlands).

Chinese translation: 一些 有着 多个 社会 保障 组织 的 卫生系 统(如 哥伦比亚、德国 及 荷兰)引入了 中央 收取 机构 来 负 责 各个 集资体 之间的 风险 公平化 _(fair sharing of risks)_.

5. Intra-pool via non-risk-related contribution and inter-pool via a _**central risk equalisation fund.**_

Chinese translation: 非风险 相关的 出资的 内部 集资 以及 集中 风险 公平性 基金 _(a risk-centralising fair fund)_.

These five textual excerpts were extracted using the English expression 'equalisation' as the search word. In the English original document, 'equalisation' appeared throughout the discussions on the importance of developing effective primary healthcare policy intervention especially in the developing world in the 1990s. The word 'equalisation' thus represents a core concept in the English source materials. Similar to the word 'risk', this was a newly introduced concept in the Chinese translation, which was to have important impact on the healthcare system reforms in mainland China (see the previous chapter on a brief review of China's healthcare system since the 1950s). Different from the word 'risk', which is largely definitional and descriptive, 'equalisation' underscores a dynamic process and sets of strategies to balance interests and minimise risks in health policy-making.

The corpus analysis of the English source text shows that high-frequency collocations of the search word 'equalisation' were 'risks', 'financial contributions', 'resources' and 'income' in the original English policy document. Given the conceptual complexity of the word 'equalisation' and related compound or multiword expressions, the translation of the original English document requires more advanced techniques to produce concise, easily understandable and consistent health translation terminologies. The parallel corpus analysis of the Chinese translation variations however reveals important variation and sometimes even confusion in the interpretation of the original English texts.

For example, in the sentence No. 2, the words '_risk and income equalisation_' was translated as 风险 公平性 及 收入 公平性 机制 (fēng xiǎn gōng píng xìng jí shōu rù gōng píng xìng jī zhì) which when translated back into English means 'the fairness of risks and a fair mechanism of incomes'. The Chinese translator had clearly reinterpreted and heavily culturally contextualised the original English expression within the socialist healthcare system at the time. The translation had in this way misled the target audience in the understanding of the original policy materials. The following two sentence pairs (No. 3 and No. 4) between the original English sentence and the Chinese translation again demonstrate the confusion caused by translating 'equalisation' with 'fairness' and 'equality'.

In No. 3, the original English expression '*equalisation for resource allocation*' was translated to Chinese as '公平的 资源 分配 机制' (gōng píng de zī yuán fēn pèi jī zhì) which means '*a fair or equitable mechanism for resource allocation*'. In No. 4, the original English expression '*risk equalisation*' was translated into 风险 公平化 (fēng xiǎn gōng píng huà) or the 'fair sharing of risks' which implies that the current distribution of (healthcare contribution) risks was not equitable or fair. The original English document suggested and described a new risk distribution strategy that was being implemented around the world (Colombia, Germany and the Netherlands), rather than the fairness, or the lack of it, of the risks related to healthcare contribution.

Another typical example of the complexity entailed in the translation of health policy technical terms is No. 5. In this sentence, the English source expression '*central risk equalisation fund*' was translated to '集中 风险 公平性 基金' (ií zhòng fēng xiǎn gong píng xìng jī jīn) which means a 'risk-centralising fair fund' in Chinese. Whereas these are arguable and controversial translations of the original source text expressions, the parallel corpus analysis detected and subsequently extracted more valid variant translations that suggested more acceptable translation strategies. These variant translations will be analysed using corpus methodologies such as word collocation and distributional patterns in the next chapter of the book.

CONCEPTUAL CLUSTER: CAPITATION

1. There are, however, a few instances in the world where attempts have been made to separate the functions and allocate resources from a pooling organisation to multiple purchasers through *__risk-adjusted capitation__*.

   Chinese translation: 但是, 世界上 也有 一些 少数的 例子 做出 努力 将 这 两项 功能 分离 并 将 资金 由 集资组织 通过 风险调整 的 人头税 (tong guò fēng xiǎn tiáo zhěng de rén tóu shuì) *(poll tax adjusted by risks)* 分配 给 多个 购买方。

2. Providers can play a role as pooling organisations under a *non-risk-adjusted capitation payment mechanism*, as discussed above. Chinese translation: 如上所述, 在 非风险调整 人头税 的支付机制 *(fēi fēng xiǎn tiáo zhěng rén tóu shuì de zhī fù jīzhì) (poll tax payment mechanism which is not adjusted by risks)* 中, 卫生 干预 措施 的 提供方 可以 扮演 如同 集资组织 的 角色。

These last two examples under the conceptual cluster 'capitation' illustrate and perhaps offer possible explanations for the detected terminological variation and sometime inconsistency in the Chinese translation of WHO health policy materials. In the first example, the word 'capitation' was translated to an existing Chinese idiom (*rén tóu shuì, poll or head tax*), a culturally loaded expression abundant in specialised Chinese domestic taxation policy materials. The Chinese translation implicitly replaced or *domesticated* the intended semantic meaning of the English original expression which represents important public health financing strategies. The result of the Chinese health translation was thus closely linked to a type of heavily culturally contextualised taxation practice in China. The original English expression 'capitation' which included both the allocation of resources (No. 1) and the collection of healthcare payments (No. 2) was culturally interpreted and adapted as *poll or head tax.*

This translation strategy may well have impacted on the reception of the original document among the target audiences, and more importantly, the subsequent development and reform of healthcare policy in the target cultural and social system that the translation was intended for. It was found in earlier studies on the impact of WHO health policy translation on national health policy that the high-quality health policy translation played a key and instrumental role in national health administration reforms and related public health legislation. A typical example is the Japanese translation and public release of the key WHO health policy document on drinking water quality guidelines in 2004 which had significant impact on the systematic reforms of the Japanese drinking water management systems and infrastructure both at national and local levels.

In Japan, standardisation of drinking water quality forms a key procedure in the development of national health policy coherent with guidelines from international health agencies such as the World Health Organisation (WHO). Policy documents such as the WHO Drinking Water Quality Guidelines form an authoritative basis for the setting of national regulations and standards for water safety in support of public health. In Japan, the Waterworks Ordinance (the 'old Waterworks Act') of 1890 did not include provisions for drinking water quality standards (DWQS). In 1908, the Council on Waterworks laid down the 'Agreed Method of Water Examination' as the national standard method for inspecting water quality.

In 1958, the DWQS were established based on the Waterworks Act, which was enacted in the previous year. After minor amendments in 1960, 1966 and 1978, the standards went through a substantial amendment in 1992. When the Waterworks Act was enacted in 1958, 29 items were set as the first DWQS. Since then, the Ministry of Health made a series of amendments on the standards to comply with the latest scientific knowledge. Among those amendments, the one conducted in 1992 was especially significant. The standard items were increased from 26 to 46 in order to substantially enhance drinking water quality management.

In 2002, in response to the WHO Third Guidelines of Drinking Water Quality, the Japanese Ministry of Health, Labour and Welfare (MHLW) consulted with the Health Science Council on the revision of DWQS in Japan. Special task forces were formed to discuss the revision of the water quality management systems. In 2004, new standards and the water quality management systems were formed and went into effect in the same year as the WHO published its Third Guidelines. The first and second editions of the WHO Guidelines for Drinking water Quality were used by developing and developed countries as the basis for regulation and standard setting to ensure the safety of drinking water.

The third edition of the Guidelines was comprehensively updated to take account of developments in risk assessment and risk management since the second edition. It described a framework for drinking water safety and discussed the roles and responsibilities of different stakeholders, including the complementary roles of national regulators, suppliers, communities and independent surveillance agencies. Developments in the third edition of the Guidelines included firstly, expanded guidance on drinking water quality management, in particular through comprehensive system-specific water safety plans. Secondly, recognizing the need for different tools and approaches in supporting large and community supplies, the third edition described the principal characteristics of the approaches to each, and the surveillance of small community supplies.

These two WHO Guidelines principles were fully represented in the revision of DWQS in Japan in 2004. Before this amendment, the DWQS were set only for items that are commonly seen throughout the nation as cause of the problems. For problems that are seen only locally or in the specific water purification methods, governmental instructions were made as a form of administrative guidance. In the amendment, such principles were reconsidered, and new standards were established based on the two fundamental principles closely in line with the Third WHO Guidelines.

Firstly, the standards were set for all items that have the possibility to cause an adverse effect on human health or living condition regardless of the locality, types of water sources, or purification methods, even if the detection level of these items is low on a national basis. Secondly, water management authorities were obliged to carry out drinking water quality examination. To make their examination appropriate and transparent, the new system required each water management authority to prepare 'Annual Water Quality Examination Plan' that indicates the boundaries for analysis, and to publish their plans for water consumers beforehand.

Fukumoto and Ji (2016) first constructed a parallel Japanese and English database which contained the full-text Japanese translation of the original WHO document. This entailed the laborious and extremely time-consuming manual alignment at sentence and clause levels between the original English texts and the Japanese translations. After the parallel corpus construction, the two researchers developed statistical machine translation methods to extract and evaluate the quality of bilingual terminologies developed in the Japanese version of the Third WHO Guidelines of Drinking Water Quality published in 2004, the same year in which the original English policy materials were published.

The translation of international policy documents requires important significant efforts to develop specialised terminologies which can convey both international scientific and policy principles in linguistic expressions that can be construed and accepted by national audiences. The empirical result showed that despite the range of new scientific knowledge especially health safety standards and newly introduced water management instruments like Water Safety Plan (WSP) which were abundant in the Third WHO Guidelines of DWQ, the Japanese translation exhibited high-level consistency. This was particularly challenging in the early 2000s when large-scale digital resources like corpora and modern translation technologies such as translation memory or statistical machine translation were at an early stage of development.

The WSP was a management tool through which the WHO introduced a comprehensive risk assessment and management approach encompassing all steps in water supplies. Following the 2004 translation, the Ministry of Health compiled the Japanese version of the guidelines which were delivered to drinking water managements across Japan in 2008.

The two case studies were based on two full-text Chinese and Japanese official translations of key WHO health policy materials around similar periods, i.e. the late 1990s and the early 2000s. This was a period before the availability of online translation aids and tools afforded by rapid technological advances made in statistical machine translation and computational linguistics. Without quality research-based online translation tools and information resources which translators use and/ or consult with extensively in their assignments nowadays, the distinct approaches to international health policy translation by professional translators in the two countries became very clear and more pronounced, as these were detected and reflected in the corpus-based analysis of the two sets of translated texts.

The contrastive national studies demonstrate that quality health policy translation can have significant impact on the public understanding, sociocultural assimilation and more importantly, the subsequent adjustment of national health policies and administration approaches to align with those promoted and identified in authoritative international health policies, standards and guidelines. These studies point to and highlight the urgent and pressing needs to develop high-quality translation terminologies, relevant translation terminological standardisation frameworks, and translation quality assessment mechanisms for health translation in general, and for international and national health policy translation, in particular. This will require, as this book argues, the development of much-needed interdisciplinary health translation which combines and leverages expertise and knowledge from a range of highly specialised fields such as corpus translation studies, computational linguistics, information technology, public health, medical science and public administration.

REFERENCES

Al-Amer, R., L. Ramjan, P. Glew, M. Darwish, and Y. Salamonson. 2015. Translation of interviews from a source language to a target language: Examining issues in cross-cultural health care research. *Journal of Clinical Nursing* 24(9–10): 1151–1162.

Chen, H.C., and M.L. Ng. 1989. Semantic facilitation and translation priming effects in Chinese-English bilinguals. *Memory & Cognition* 17(4): 454–462.

Fukumoto, Fumiyo, and Meng Ji. (2016). Statistical machine translation for evaluating WHO environmental health policy translation terminology. Paper presented at the Inaugural Workshop on Empirical Translation Studies, University of Sydney, Australia.

Laviosa, Sara. 2002. *Corpus-based Translation Studies: Theory, Findings, Applications*, vol. 17. Amsterdam: Rodopi.

Olohan, Maeve. 2004. *Introducing Corpora in Translation Studies*. London: Routledge.

Shuzhang, Du. 2008. *Taxation in Imperial Chinese Societies (zhōng guó huáng quán shè huì de fù shuì yán jiū)*. Beijing: Chinese Finance and Economics Press.

Teich, E. 2003. *Cross-Linguistic Variation in System and Text: A Methodology for the Investigation of Translations and Comparable Texts*. Berlin: Walter de Gruyter.

World Health Organisation. 2000a. (Annual report) *Health systems: Improving performance*. http://www.who.int/whr/2000/en/whr00_en.pdf.

World Health Organisation. 2000b. (Annual Report), trans. *She Jie Wei Sheng Bao Gao: Wei Sheng Xi Tong Gai Jin Bao Gao*. Chinese Ministry of Health, Beijing: People's Health Press.

CHAPTER 5

A Corpus-Based Collocation Analysis of Terminological Variation in Chinese Health Translation

Abstract This chapter deploys large Chinese databases to analyse the collocation and disciplinary distribution patterns of variant Chinese translations of health terms. The corpus-based analysis compares over an extended period of time newly created health expressions with health translations adapted from or simply borrowing existing culturally conventionalised terms in Chinese formal discourses. The corpus empirical analysis suggests that culturally and linguistically localised expressions of health financial risks tend to be better construed and established in the target Chinese knowledge system. The corpus analysis of variant health risk translations also reveals that the focus and specific approaches to critical health topics such as healthcare financial risks exhibit different patterns at the international and national levels.

Keywords Collocation analysis · Chinese health translation Corpus data mining

In Chap. 4, after the construction of the English and Chinese parallel translation database, four conceptual clusters of health risks terms were extracted and selected for a close English-Chinese contrastive analysis to illustrate important lexical and terminological variations in the Chinese translation of key WHO health policy materials, i.e. the 2000 WHO global health annual report. These were 'risk factor', '(health risks or healthcare contribution) equalisation', '(risk-adjusted healthcare

© The Author(s) 2017
M. Ji, *Translation and Health Risk Knowledge Building in China*,
DOI 10.1007/978-981-10-4681-0_5

contribution) capitation' and '(health financing or healthcare) sustainability'. It was argued that translation variation detected within these conceptual or terminological clusters underscores diverse translation strategies and approaches used in the Mandarin Chinese version of the 2000 WHO health annual report on global health financial risks. The purpose of this chapter is to offer a corpus-based linguistic analysis of subtle differences between these Chinese variant translations of the English source text expressions. This offers an empirical or corpus-based exploration of the understanding and uptake of new idea sets and concepts related to healthcare risks introduced via the translation of key international health policy materials among both a general target audience and more specialised readers such as Chinese academic researchers and the media professionals.

In this process, large-scale original Chinese databases such as the CNKI database will be deployed and explored by using well-tested corpus analytical methodologies such as corpus-based word collocation analysis and word-frequency-based lexical distributional patterns (Granger and Paquot 2012; Hanks 2012a, b). While the majority of publications in the CNKI database are in original Mandarin Chinese, a growing number of the original Chinese publications are constantly and systematically translated and integrated into the database. In recent years, the research company CNKI International Publishing Centre which manages the database launched an ambitious ongoing project which coordinates a large number of academics and researchers based at Chinese and overseas institutes to contribute to the translation of original Chinese research materials in the CNKI database (Zheng and Jiang 2013). Important research investments such as the CNKI Translation Project underscore the growing demands both within and outside China for high-quality bilingual translation to facilitate the exchange of ideas and knowledge in scientific, technological, medical and social sciences across languages, cultures and societies.

For the current study, four conceptual clusters of health risks were analysed in depth (Table 5.1). Each conceptual cluster contains at least two Chinese lexical variant translations. These lexical variations are seen as translation synonyms to each other, given the high frequencies of occurrence as interchanging translations of the source English terms in the original health policy document. Their interchanging deployment in the Chinese translated document as variant translations of the original English terms by different Chinese translators implies that they point

Table 5.1 Conceptual clusters of health financial risk and intra-cluster Chinese translation variations

No	Conceptual clusters	Chinese translation variations
1.	Risk factor	1. Dangerous elements; 2. Dangerous factors; 3. Risk factor
2.	(Health risk or health financial contribution) Equalisation	1. Balancing; 2. Equalise; 3. Equalisation
3.	(Healthcare or healthcare contribution) Capitation	1. Taxation per head (poll tax or head tax) 2. Payment per capita
4.	(Healthcare financing) Sustainability	1. Sustainability; 2. Economic dynamics 3. Economic affordability

Table 5.2 Disciplinary distribution of 'dangerous elements (危险因子)' in CNKI

Disciplinary Distribution	Chinese Translation	Frequency of occurrence
心血管系统疾病	Cardiovascular disease	4665
内分泌腺及全身性疾病	Endocrine glands and systemic diseases	1805
神经病学	Neurology	1093
肿瘤学	Oncology	951
临床医学	Clinical medicine	683
急救医学	Emergency medicine	515
精神病学	Psychology	333
外科学	Surgery	323
泌尿科学	Urology	315
基础医学	Basic medicine	312

to a shared conceptual and terminological cluster in the mind of native Chinese speakers. However, subtle and important differences do exist among these variant translations in terms of their semantic meaning and usage in specific domains and areas in the Chinese language. The corpus-based analysis in this chapter will distinguish such differences among these linguistic variations based on their different collocation patterns in the CNKI database, and their distinct distribution patterns across disciplines and research fields in China.

Tables 5.2, 5.3, 5.4, 5.5, 5.6 and 5.7 exhibit the collocation patterns of the three Chinese translation variations under the conceptual cluster 'risk factor'. While the Chinese expression风险因素 (fēng xiǎn yīn

Table 5.3   Top collocates of 'dangerous elements (危险因子)' in CNKI

Chinese top collocates	Translation	Frequency of occurrence
冠心病	Coronary heart disease	997
危险因素	Dangerous elements	891
同型半胱氨酸	Homocysteine	640
高血压	Hypertension	577
糖尿病	Diabetes	448

sù, risk factor) appears to the closest translation, the other two Chinese translations 危险因素 (wéi xiǎn yīn sù, dangerous factor) and 危险因子 (wéi xiǎn yīn zǐ, dangerous element) also proved to be highly frequent translation variations of the original English expression 'risk factor'. In fact, all of the three translation variations displayed consistent patterns which suggested a strong cross-lingual semantic matching and alignment emerged in the parallel translation corpus analysis. A close linguistic analysis of the differences among these expressions is thus necessary. Semantic disambiguation between linguistic synonyms in the same language has been explored using corpus resources, tools and methodologies successfully and productively. This study will introduce and adapt this established corpus analysis methodology for the study of translation synonyms. That is, the semantic differentiation among variant translations will be based on their word collocation and distributional patterns in the large-scale Chinese reference corpus used.

Conceptual Cluster of 'Risk Factor' and Associated Chinese Expressions
(1) 危险因子 (dangerous element); (2) 危险因素 (dangerous factor); (3) 风险因素 (risk factor)

Tables 5.2 and 5.3 show the top collocates of the term 'dangerous elements' (危险因子) as a variant translation of the English word 'risk factor'. The top collocates include 'coronary heart disease' (997); 'dangerous factors' (891); 'homo-cysteinaemia' (640); 'high blood pressure' (577) and 'diabetes' (448). Numbers in brackets indicate the frequencies of occurrence of the collocated expressions to the variant translation in the Chinese reference corpus which was used to examine the use of these variant translations in the original Chinese language. This helps to identify and explore the dynamic textual context in which the target audience or the Chinese readers tend to understand and interpret the semantic

Table 5.4 Disciplinary distribution of 'dangerous factors (危险因素)' in CHKI

Disciplinary Distribution	Chinese Translation	Frequency of occurrence
心血管系统疾病	Cardiovascular disease	26,162
临床医学	Clinical medicine	15,936
神经病学	Neurology	15,897
内分泌腺及全身性疾病	Endocrine glands and systemic diseases	15,393
肿瘤学	Oncology	10,830
预防医学与卫生学	Preventative medicine and hygiene	8982
外科学	Surgery	8523
妇产科学	Obstetrics and gynaecology	6487
儿科学	Paediatrics	6309
急救医学	Emergency medicine	5590

Table 5.5 Top collocates of 'dangerous factors (危险因素)' in CNKI

Chinese top collocates	Translation	Frequency of occurrence
高血压	Hypertension	6521
糖尿病	Diabetes	5056
预后	Prognosis	4226
冠心病	Coronary heart disease	4173
影响因素	Influencing factors	3733

meaning of the translated terms. Tables 5.4 and 5.5 reveal that in the CNKI database, the top collocates of the variant translation 'dangerous factors (危险因素)' are 'high blood pressure' (6521); 'diabetes' (5056); 'prognosis' (4226); 'coronary heart disease' (4173) and 'influencing or explanatory factor' (3733).

Tables 5.6 and 5.7 show that the top collocates of the variant translation 'risk factor' (风险因素) are 'risk' (3531), 'risk administration' (3075), 'dangerous factor' (2596), 'influencing or explanatory factor' (2146) and 'risk assessment or evaluation' (1754). There are some overlaps in the collocation patterns among the three variant translations, for example, 'dangerous factors (危险因素)' have proved to be the top collocate of both variant translations 'dangerous elements' (危险因子) and 'risk factor' (风险因素); and 'influencing or explanatory factor' was detected as one of the top collocates for both variant translations

Table 5.6   Disciplinary distribution of 'risk factors (风险因素)' in CHKI

Disciplinary Distribution	Chinese Translation	Frequency of occurrence
金融	Finance	11,347
企业经济	Business economy	8919
宏观经济管理和可持续发展	Macro-economic management and sustainable development	7963
投资	Investment	7230
临床医学	Clinical medicine	5319
肿瘤学	Oncology	4200
工业经济	Industry economy	4052
心血管系统疾病	Cardiovascular disease	2890
证券	Securities	2814
内分泌腺及全身性疾病	Endocrine glands and systemic diseases	2343

Table 5.7   Top collocates of 'risk factors (风险因素)' in CNKI

Chinese top collocates	Translation	Frequency of occurrence
风险	Risks	3531
风险管理	Risk management	3075
危险因素	Dangerous elements	2596
影响因素	Influencing elements	2146
风险评估	Risk assessment	1754

'dangerous factors (危险因素)' and 'risk factor' (风险因素). However, distinct collocation patterns did emerge from the corpus analysis which brought insights into the semantic differences among the variant Chinese translations of the English word 'risk factor'.

The corpus analysis identified important collocation patterns that assist us with the disambiguation of the semantic and usage differences among these terms in original Chinese. Firstly, the corpus patterns show that the first two Chinese variants translations 'dangerous elements' (危险因子) and 'dangerous factors (危险因素)' are more frequently used in specialised medical and health domains. This was established in their top collocates detected in the corpus analysis which suggest strong semantic links

Table 5.8 Disciplinary distribution of '*Equalise* (均衡)' in CHKI

Disciplinary Distribution	Chinese Translation	Frequency of occurrence
宏观经济管理与可持续发展	Macro-economic management and sustainable development	24,947
金融	Finance	14,636
经济体制改革	Economic system reform	14,242
数学	Maths	8953
企业经济	Business economy	8806
电信技术	Telecommunication technology	8621
教育理论与教育管理	Educational theory and educational management	8303
投资	Investment	7090
农业经济	Agricultural economy	6623
经济理论与经济思想史	Economic theory and history	6470

between these variant translations with specialised health terms such as 'cardiovascular diseases', 'high blood pressure' and 'diabetes'. Secondly, the third Chinese variant translation 'risk factor' (风险因素) which is suggested by most dictionaries as the closest Chinese translation of the English source expression displayed a set of very different collocation patterns. The corpus analysis reveals that the Chinese word 风险因素 is more frequently used in specialised domains such as finance, economics, business and management, as the top collocates of the word are 'risk administration', 'influencing or explanatory factor' and 'risk assessment or evaluation'.

Conceptual Cluster of '(health risk) Equalisation' and Associated Chinese Expressions
(1) 均衡 (Equalise); (2) 平衡 (balance); (3) 均衡化 (equalisation)

Tables 5.8, 5.9, 5.10, 5.11, 5.12 and 5.13 exhibit the collocation patterns of the three Chinese variant translations within the conceptual cluster '(health risk or healthcare contribution) equalisation'. The closest Chinese translation of the English source text expression is '*equalisation* (均衡化 jūn héng huà)', but the other two Chinese expressions 'equalise (均衡 jūn héng)' and 'balance (平衡 píng héng)' have also been identified in the parallel corpus analysis as alternative translations of the original English expression '*equalisation* (均衡化 jūn héng huà)'.

Tables 5.8 and 5.9 show that in the CNKI database the top collocates of the expression 'equalise (均衡 jūn héng)' are 'load-equalising' (2893); 'economic growth' (2778); 'board game (Chinese chess)' (2528);

Table 5.9   Top collocates of '*Equalise* (均衡)' in CNKI

Chinese top collocates	Translation	Frequency of occurrence
负载均衡	Load-equalising	2893
经济增长	Economic growth	2778
博弈	Board game	2528
均衡	EQUALISE	2366
博弈论	Game theories	1870

Table 5.10   Disciplinary distribution of '*Balance* (平衡)' in CHKI

Disciplinary Distribution	Chinese Translation	Frequency of occurrence
电力工业	Electricity industry	25,777
建筑科学与工程	Architecture and engineering	20,525
经济体制改革	Economic system reform	19,502
金融	Finance	18,705
农业经济	Agricultural economy	18,012
宏观经济管理与可持续发展	Macro-economic management and sustainable development	17,505
企业经济	Business economy	17,173
环境科学与资源利用	Environmental science and resource utilisation	17,061
工业经济	Industrial economy	16,361
化学	Chemistry	15,285

'equalise' (2366) and 'game theories' (1870). Tables 5.10 and 5.11 shows the top collocates of the expression 'balance (平衡 píng héng)' are 'adsorption' (4359); 'stability' (3564); 'countermeasures' (3545); 'balanced scorecard' (3167); and 'health care' (2266). Tables 5.12 and 5.13 show the top collocates of the expression 'equalisation (均衡化 jūn héng huà)' are 'image enhancement' (434); 'histogram equalisation' (285); 'image processing' (178); 'equalisation' (155) and 'mandatory education' (100).

The disciplinary distributions of these three expressions match the collocation patterns. In Table 5.8, the ten Chinese subjects or research areas which have produced substantial publications on 'equalise (均衡 jūn héng)' are macro-economic management and sustainable growth

Table 5.11   Top collocates of '*Balance* (平衡)' in CNKI

Chinese top collocates	Translation	Frequency of occurrence
吸附	Adsorption	4359
稳定性	Stability	3564
对策	Counter measures	3545
平衡记分卡	Balanced scorecard	3167
护理	Care	2266

Table 5.12   Disciplinary distribution of '*equalisation* (均衡化)' in CHKI

Disciplinary Distribution	Chinese Translation	Frequency of occurrence
计算机软件及计算机应用	Computer software and application	1444
教育理论与教育管理	Educational theory and management	611
中等教育	Secondary education	187
经济体制改革	Economic system reform	158
宏观经济管理与可持续发展	Macro-economic management and sustainable development	137
自动化技术	Automation technology	124
高等教育	Higher education	96
农业经济	Agricultural economy	95
中国政治与国际政治	Chinese politics and international politics	84
电信技术	Telecommunication technology	76

Table 5.13   Top collocates of '*equalisation* (均衡化)' in CNKI

Chinese top collocates	Translation	Frequency of occurrence
图像增强	Image enhancement	434
直方图均衡化	Histogram equalisation	285
图像处理	Image processing	178
均衡化	Equalisation	155
义务教育	Compulsory education	100

(24,947); finance (14,636); economic system reform (14,242); maths (8953); corporate economy (8808); telecommunication (8621); education theory and management (8303); investment (7090); agricultural economy (6623) and economic theories and history of economic thoughts (6470). Similar to the collocation patterns of the word 'equalise (均衡 jūn héng)', the disciplinary distribution points to the strong link of this linguistic expression with the study of economy and finance in the target language and social context.

In Table 5.10, the ten Chinese subjects or research areas which have yielded the largest numbers of publications on 'balance (平衡 píng héng)' are electric power industry (25,777); architecture and architectural engineering (20,525); economic system reform (19,502); finance (18,705); agricultural economy (18,012); macro-economic management and sustainable growth (17,505); corporate economy (17,173); environmental science and resources use (17,061); industrial economy (16,361); chemistry (15,285). The disciplinary distribution matches the collocation patterns of the word 'balance (平衡 píng héng)'. Compared with the word 'equalise (均衡 jūn héng)', the word 'balance (平衡 píng héng)' appears to be more general, as it has occurred not only in economic subject areas but also in electric power industry, architecture, environmental science and chemistry.

In Table 5.12, the top subject or research area which has featured the word 'equalisation (均衡化 jūn héng huà)' is computer software and application (1444) which accounts for almost half of the entire publications having the word 'equalisation (均衡化 jūn héng huà)' as the keyword. The second largest research area in which the word 'equalisation (均衡化 jūn héng huà)' reoccurs is education theory and management (611)—this area accounts for nearly a quarter of the total publications on the topic of 'equalisation (均衡化 jūn héng huà)'. The remaining relevant subject fields include secondary education (187); economic system reform (158); macro-economic management and sustainable growth (137); automation technology (124); higher education (96); agricultural economy (95); Chinese and international politics (84) and telecommunication (76). The distribution statistics reveal that apart from the computer science and software engineering, the word 'equalisation (均衡化 jūn héng huà)' has distinctively different distributions in Chinese academic publications from its lemma 'equalise (均衡 jūn héng)' (see Fig. 6.1).

The noun which refers to a changing process as indicated by its suffix '-tion' has a wider and diversified application in Chinese research fields especially in the social sciences such as education, politics, apart from sub-branches of economics. It is worthwhile noticing that despite the word 'equalisation (均衡化 jūn héng huà)' is the closest linguistic translation of the English source expression, matching between the two words across languages entails an important shift in the genre distribution of the Chinese word, which might potentially cause the discipline-based (mis-)understanding of the translation word by specialised and/or general audiences.

Conceptual Cluster of 'Sustainability' and Associated Chinese Expressions

1. 可持续性 *(kě chí xù xìng, sustainability)*
2. 经济活力 *(jīng jì huó lì, economic dynamics)*
3. 经济承受能力 *(jīng jì chéng shòu néng lì, economic affordability)*

Tables 5.14, 5.15, 5.16, 5.17, 5.18 and 5.19 display the collocation patterns of the three Chinese variant translations within the conceptual cluster '(health financing) sustainability'. The word 'sustainability' (可持续性 kě chí xù xìng) appears to the nearest translation of the English word. The expressions 'economic dynamics' (经济活力 jīng jì huó lì) and 'economic affordability' (经济承受能力 jīng jì chéng shòu néng lì) proved to be, as the CNKI database shows, closely related to the word 'sustainability' (可持续性 kě chí xù xìng) conceptually, as academics and translators alternated the use of these three words in different textual contexts touching upon the topic of financial sustainability.

Table 5.15 shows that the top collocates of the word 'sustainability' (可持续性 kě chí xù xìng) in the CNKI database which are 'sustainable development' (2382); 'sustainability' (580); 'economic growth' (404); 'countermeasures' (372) and 'circular economy' (336). Table 5.17 shows that the top collocates of the word 'economic dynamics' (经济活力 jīng jì huó lì) are 'countermeasures' (572); 'small- and medium-sized enterprises' (SMSE) (530); 'development' (413); 'innovation' (386) and 'problems' (280).

Table 5.19 shows that the top collocates of the word 'economic affordability' (经济承受能力 jīng jì chéng shòu néng lì) are 'countermeasures' (39); 'affordability' (29); 'rural areas' (18); 'problems' (17)

Table 5.14 Disciplinary distribution of '*sustainability* (可持续性)' in CHKI

Disciplinary Distribution	Chinese Translation	Frequency of occurrence
宏观经济管理与可持续发展	Macro-economic management and sustainable development	3601
经济体制改革	Economic system reform	3109
农业经济	Agricultural economy	2077
环境科学与资源利用	Environmental science and resource utilisation	1773
工业经济	Industrial economy	1389
企业经济	Business economy	1102
金融	Finance	975
建筑科学与工程	Architecture and engineering	861
经济理论与经济思想史	Economic theory and history	661
资源科学	Resource science	659

Table 5.15 Top collocates of '*sustainability* (可持续性)' in CNKI

Chinese top collocates	Translation	Frequency of occurrence
可持续发展	Sustainable development	2382
可持续性	Sustainability	580
经济增长	Economic growth	404
对策	Countermeasures	372
循环经济	Circular economy	336

and 'social security' (16). The collocation patterns seem to suggest that the word 'sustainability' (可持续性 kě chí xù xìng) is strongly associated with the development of new economic models to stimulate economic growth in China. On the other hand, the word 'economic dynamics' (经济活力 jīng jì huó lì) is closely tied with the internal economic reforms within China in which small- and medium-sized enterprises (SMSE) and innovation are seen as two key factors and driving forces to inject more dynamics into the national economy. Lastly, the word 'economic affordability' (经济承受能力 jīng jì chéng shòu néng lì) appears to be linked to social problems in rural China which include among others, the welfare and social security of people living in remote rural areas (Long et al. 2013; Gong et al. 2012; Meng et al. 2015).

A close look at the disciplinary distribution patterns of these three words confirm the findings emerged in the collocation analysis. In Table 5.14, the top three research areas which have produced the largest publications on 'sustainability' are macro-economic management and sustainable growth (3601); economic system reform (3109) and agricultural economy (2077). These are followed by environmental science and resources use (1773); industrial economy (1389); corporate economy (1102); finance (975); architecture and architectural engineering (861); economic theories and history of economic thoughts (661) and resources science (659).

The distribution patterns of the word 'sustainability' (可持续性) reveal important findings regarding how the development of new economic models unfolds in China as evidenced in sustained academic publications collected in the CNKI database. Apart from macro-economic management and reform to environmental and resources sciences, the word 'sustainability' (可持续性) underscores the multidimensional social and economic transition that China has undergone and continues to push through in the next few decades (Tilt 2013; Zhang et al. 2013; Ma et al. 2015). It can thus be expected that the word 'sustainability' (可持续性) will develop new dimensions of meaning as it is used in growing and emerging research areas built around sustainability.

Table 5.16 shows that the top two research areas which account for almost half of the total publications on 'economic dynamics' (经济活力) are corporate economy (9509) and economic system reform (7729). These areas are followed by industrial economy (3402); agricultural economy (3115); macro-economic management and sustainable growth (2945); finance (2882); trade economy (1694); Chinese and international politics (1523); higher education (1350) and Chinese Communist Party (1235). The distribution patterns of the word 'economic dynamics' (经济活力) indicate that this word is strongly associated with Chinese internal economic reforms and to some extent, its internal political agenda. The use of this word can therefore trigger in the native Chinese speakers' mind the drastic economic reforms across corporates, the industrial and agricultural sectors, finance and trade in China since the early 1980s (Du and Yang 2014; Cao and Birchenall 2013).

In Table 5.18, the top three disciplinary areas that have produced the most academic publications on 'economic affordability' are agricultural

Table 5.16   Disciplinary distribution of '*Economic dynamics* (经济活力)' in CHKI

Disciplinary Distribution	Chinese Translation	Frequency of occurrence
企业经济	Business economy	9509
经济体制改革	Economic system reform	7729
工业经济	Industrial economy	3402
农业经济	Agricultural economy	3115
宏观经济管理与可持续性发展	Macro-economic management and sustainable development	2945
金融	Finance	2882
贸易经济	Trade economy	1694
中国政治与国际政治	Chinese and international politics	1523
高等教育	Higher education	1350
中国共产党	Chinese communist party	1235

Table 5.17   Top collocates of '*Economic dynamics* (经济活力)' in CNKI

Chinese top collocates	Translation	Frequency of occurrence
对策	Countermeasures	572
中小企业	Small and medium-sized businesses	530
发展	Development	413
创新	Innovation	386
问题	Problems	280

economy (426); macro-economic management and sustainable growth (228) and investment (180). These areas are followed by a number of research areas which have seen a limited number of research publications discussing the issue: medicine and health guidelines, policies, laws and regulations (106); higher education (90); industrial economy (87); trade economy (84); economic system reform (77); finance and taxation (75) and insurance (62). This finding complements the collocation patterns of the word 'economic affordability' (经济承受能力). This word is chiefly linked with social and economic problems in rural China.

Table 5.18 Disciplinary distribution of '*Economic affordability*' (经济承受能力) in CHKI

Disciplinary Distribution	Chinese Translation	Frequency of occurrence
农业经济	Agricultural economy	426
宏观经济管理与可持续发展	Macro-economic management and sustainable development	228
投资	Investment	180
医药卫生方针政策与法律法规研究	Research in the policy and laws and regulations of medicine and health	106
高等教育	Higher education	90
工业经济	Industrial economy	87
贸易经济	Trade economy	84
经济体制改革	Economic system reforms	77
财政与税收	Finance and taxation	75
保险	Insurance	62

Table 5.19 Top collocates of '*Economic affordability*' (经济承受能力) in CNKI

Chinese top collocates	Translation	Frequency of occurrence
对策	Countermeasures	39
承受能力	Affordability	29
农村	Rural areas	18
问题	Problems	17
社会保障	Social security	16

Conceptual Cluster of '(Risk-Adjusted) Capitation' and Associated Chinese Expressions

1: 人头税 *(Taxation per head/poll tax)* 2: 按人头付费 *(payment per capita)*

Tables 5.20, 5.21, 5.22 and 5.23 display the distinct collocation patterns of the Chinese linguistic variations in the conceptual cluster '(Risk-Adjusted) Capitation' extracted from the WHO 2000 Annual Report. In Table 5.22, top collocates of the word 'taxation per head or per capita' (人头税) are 'taxation based on land ownership' (in classical Chinese; feudal Chinese tax system) (5); 'taxation' (in classical Chinese) (5); 'currency-based taxation' (twice a year) (5) (in classical Chinese, feudal

Table 5.20   Disciplinary distribution of 'Tax per head (人头税)' in CHKI

Disciplinary Distribution	Chinese Translation	Frequency of occurrence
财政与税收	Finance and taxation	58
中国古代史	Ancient Chinese history	38
中国政治与国际政治	Chinese and international politics	10
世界历史	World history	7
中国通史	History of China	6
经济体制改革	Economic system reform	4
农业经济	Agricultural economy	4
考古	Archaeology	4
贸易经济	Trade economy	3
投资	Investment	3

Table 5.21   Top collocates of 'Tax per head (人头税)' in CNKI

Chinese top collocates	Translation	Frequency of occurrence
摊丁入亩	Taxation based on land ownership	5
赋税	Taxation (in classical Chinese)	5
两税法	Currency-based taxation (in classical Chinese)	5
汉代	Han Dynasty	5
户赋	Household-based taxation	4

Chinese tax system); 'Han Dynasty' (202 B.C.–220 A.D.) (5) and 'household-based taxation' (in classical Chinese; feudal Chinese tax system) (4). By contrast, the top collocates of the word 'Payment per capita (按人头付费)' are 'payment methods' (14); 'health insurance' (11); 'new rural cooperative health care' (6); 'community health services' (5); and 'health care costs' (5).

The co-existence of the two Chinese linguistic variations for the concept of (risk-adjusted) capitation points to another important dimension of health translation in particular, and specialised translation in general, i.e. the use of existing domain-specific idioms and technical jargons in the target language. A close inspection of the source text shows that neither of the two Chinese linguistic variations has fully conveyed

Table 5.22 Disciplinary distribution of 'Payment per capita (按人头付费)' in CHKI

Disciplinary Distribution	Chinese Translation	Frequency of occurrence
医药卫生方针政策与法律法规研究	Research in the policy and laws and regulations of medicine and health	90
保险	Insurance	53
投资	Investment	37
药学	Pharmacy	4
医学教育与医学边缘科学	Medical education and medical edge science	2
特种医学	Medical aspects of harsh environments	2
军事医学与卫生	Military medicine and health	2
农业经济	Agricultural economy	1
工业经济	Industrial economy	1
财政与税收	Finance and taxation	1

Table 5.23 Top collocates of 'Payment per capita (按人头付费)' in CNKI

Chinese top collocates	Translation	Frequency of occurrence
支付方式	Payment method	14
医疗保险	Medical insurance	11
新型农村合作医疗	New rural cooperative medical care	6
社区卫生服务	Community health services	5
医疗费用	Medical costs	5

the meaning of the original English word which refers to 'a fixed payment per beneficiary to a provider responsible for delivering a range of services' (WHO 2000 Annual Report). The use of either of the two Chinese linguistic variations can cause misunderstanding of the original health policy documents. It is therefore likely that new linguistic variations or translation versions will emerge as more academic research in China delves into the area.

REFERENCES

Cao, K.H., and J.A. Birchenall. 2013. Agricultural productivity, structural change, and economic growth in post-reform China. *Journal of Development Economics* 104:165–180.

Du, Y., and C. Yang. 2014. Demographic Transition and Labour Market Changes: Implications for Economic Development in China. *Journal of Economic Surveys* 28 (4): 617–635.

Gong, P., S. Liang, E.J. Carlton, Q. Jiang, J. Wu, L. Wang, and J.V. Remais. 2012. Urbanisation and Health in China. *The Lancet* 379 (9818): 843–852.

Granger, Sylviane, and Magali Paquot, (eds.). 2012. *Electronic Lexicography*. Oxford: Oxford University Press.

Hanks, Patrick. 2012a. Corpus Evidence and Electronic Lexicography. In *Electronic Lexicography*, eds. Granger, Sylviane and Magali Paquot. Oxford University Press.

Hanks, Patrick. 2012b. Lexicography. In Ruslan Mitkov, *Oxford Handbook of Computational Linguistics*, ed. (2nd). OUP.

Long, Q., L. Xu, H. Bekedam, and S. Tang. 2013. Changes in Health Expenditures in China in 2000s: Has the Health System Reform Improved Affordability. *International Journal for Equity in Health* 12 (1): 40.

Ma, R., L. Huang, D. Zhao, and L. Xu. 2015. Commercial Health Insurance—A New Power to Push China Healthcare Reform Forward? *Value in Health* 18 (3): A103.

Meng, Q., H. Fang, X. Liu, B. Yuan, and J. Xu. 2015. Consolidating the Social Health Insurance Schemes in China: Towards an Equitable and Efficient Health System. *The Lancet* 386 (10002): 1484–1492.

Tilt, B. 2013. *The Struggle for Sustainability in Rural China: Environmental Values and Civil Society*. New York: Columbia University Press.

World Health Organisation. 2000. *Health Systems: Improving Performance* (Annual Report). Available at http://www.who.int/whr/2000/en/whr00_en.pdf.

Zhang, X., Y. Xiong, J. Ye, Z. Deng, and X. Zhang. 2013. Analysis of Government Investment in Primary Healthcare Institutions to Promote Equity During the Three-year Health Reform Program in China. *BMC Health Services Research* 13 (1): 1.

Zheng, Q., and Jiang, S. 2013. An online Chinese-English academic dictionary based on bilingual literature abstracts. In *Information Science and Technology (ICIST) 2013 International Conference on 23 March 2013* (pp. 777–779). IEEE.

Corpus Exploration of Variant Health Translation Terms

Abstract Chapter 6 provides a corpus-based exploration of the distribution of health translations using a trend analysis and the subsequent statistical modelling of variant health translations in Chinese research publication. It was found that health terms which form the culturally adapted translation group occurred much more frequently in Chinese research publications, when compared to entirely newly created translations or word-by-word literal translations without adequate cultural and linguistic adaptation. Chapter 6 utilises statistical measures produced by large-scale databases to develop useful indicators for the study of the patterns of the distribution of health translation variants in the target language and social context.

Keywords Corpus distribution · Descriptive statistics Variant translations

6.1 DISTRIBUTIONAL ANALYSIS OF VARIANT HEALTH RISK TERMS IN CHINESE PUBLICATIONS

While linguistic analyses such as collocation patterns reveal subtle semantic differences between synonyms, they do not show the differences among these words in terms of their distribution in research publications and formal media materials over the years in China. Without such critical information, it would be difficult to assess how the deliberate or

© The Author(s) 2017   71
M. Ji, *Translation and Health Risk Knowledge Building in China*,
DOI 10.1007/978-981-10-4681-0_6

undeliberate use of linguistic variations as alternative translations may impact the outreach and wide dissemination of international health documents in national contexts. As explained from the outset of this study, the hypothesised high-performance linguistic variations tend to have a wider and sustained distribution in academic and media materials in the target language; whereas low-performance linguistic variations tend to exhibit a limited distribution in the target society which hinders the social impact and outreach of the source materials translated.

The analysis of the distribution properties of these two groups of linguistic variations, i.e. alternative translations of source text words, is based on the three quantitative measures, which are the Academic Growth Rate (AGR), academic dissemination rate (ADR) and media distribution rate (MDR) of target linguistic expressions. In this section, we will have a close look at the distribution of component linguistic expressions in four conceptual clusters. For this purpose, we used the CNKI database. Given the structure of CNKI, the study of the dissemination patterns of translated WHO public health documents in Chinese media is limited to printed media materials only.

Figure 6.1 illustrates the growth patterns of academic publications on each of the three component expressions of the conceptual cluster 'risk factor'. On the graph, there are two sets of trend lines: the upper part of the graph displays three trend lines with shadows and the lower part with three trend lines without shadows. These indicate the total numbers of

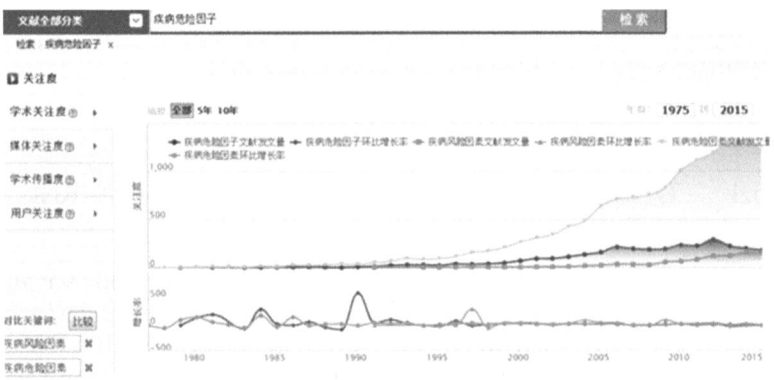

Fig. 6.1 AGR: Distribution patterns of Chinese linguistic variations of 'Risk Factor' in CNKI

academic publications on 'disease dangerous factor' (red); 'disease dangerous element' (blue) and 'disease risk factor' (yellow). For the upper part of the graph, the x-axis indicates the year of publication and the y-axis shows the publication volumes. The lower part of the graph shows the growth rate of publications on each topic, i.e. 'disease dangerous factor'; 'disease dangerous element' and 'disease risk factor'.

Figure 6.1 shows that among the three linguistic variations of the conceptual cluster 'risk factor', 'dangerous factor' and 'dangerous element' appear in Chinese academic publications much earlier than the expression 'risk factor' which was documented in the CNKI database after the early 1990s. Whereas the use of 'dangerous element' saw two surges in the 1980s and the 1990s, the distribution of the word 'dangerous factor' increased rapidly since the 1990s and the general trend of the increasing use of 'dangerous factor' compared to the other two expressions, i.e. 'dangerous element' and 'risk factor' became more noticeable after the 2000s. The trend analysis shows in terms of AGR (Academic Growth Rate); 'dangerous factor' clearly belongs to the high-performance category, whereas 'dangerous element' and 'risk factor' seem to be associated with limited amounts of academic publications over the last 20 years or so.

Figure 6.2 shows the media publications on the three components of the conceptual cluster 'risk factor'. Similar to Fig. 6.1, Fig. 6.2 is divided into two parts: the upper part shows three trend lines with shadows which are the total amount of media publication on each topic; and the

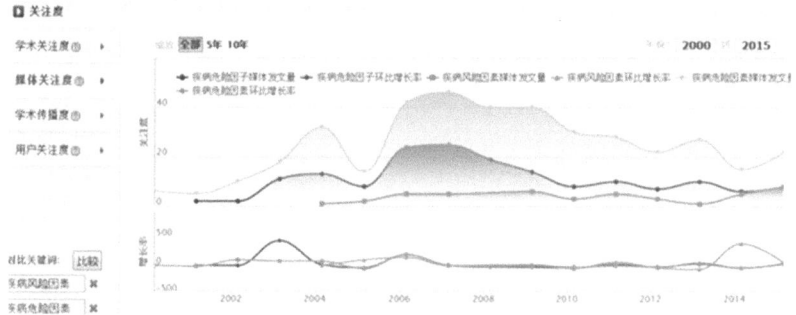

Fig. 6.2 MDR: Distribution patterns of Chinese linguistic variations of 'Risk Factor' in CNKI

lower part displays the growth rate of media publications associated with each topic or linguistic variation of 'risk factor'. The two graphs show very different patterns which suggest that Chinese media and academic publications have different focuses and priorities on the reporting and research of risk topics. Firstly, whereas in Fig. 6.1, 'disease dangerous factor' shows a rapid and accelerated growth since the 1990s, in Fig. 6.2, the media reporting of 'disease dangerous factor' reached the first peak in 2004 but it fell quickly around 2005. The media interest in this topic picked up again in 2006, continued to grow in 2007 and then gradually fell again around 2008, a general decreasing trend until recently.

Secondly, in terms of the word 'disease dangerous element', its distribution pattern in the media is comparable to that of the word 'disease dangerous factor'. This is very different from its distribution in Chinese academic publications, as only a very limited number of Chinese research publications focus on 'disease dangerous element' when compared to 'disease dangerous factor'. Thirdly, the word 'risk factor' remains low profile in both Chinese academic and media publications within the timespan investigated. The findings in Figs. 6.1 and 6.2 seem to suggest 'disease dangerous element' and 'disease dangerous factor' are high-performance linguistic variations in the media, whereas 'disease risk factor' remains a low performance word in both academic and media publications.

Figure 6.3 shows the academic cross-citation of the three component expressions of the conceptual cluster 'risk factor'. It shows that the cross reference of these linguistic variations in Chinese academic publications resemble and accentuate the picture in Fig. 6.1, i.e. the growth

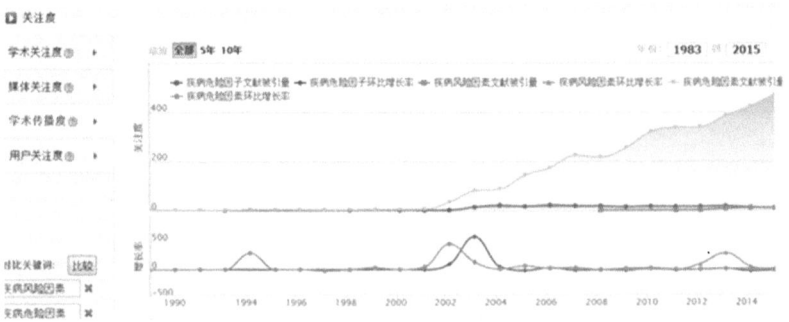

Fig. 6.3 ADR: Distribution patterns of Chinese linguistic variations of 'Risk Factor' in CNKI

Table 6.1 Comparison of variant translations of 'Risk Factor' in Chinese research and media publication

Quantitative measures	Disease dangerous factor	Disease dangerous element	Disease risk factor (3)
Academic Growth Rate (AGR)	High	Low	Low
Academic Dissemination Rate (ADR)	High	Low	Low
Media Dissemination Rate (MDR)	High	Medium	Low

rate of academic publications on each of the three topics and linguistic variations. The resemblance between Figs. 6.1 and 6.3 seems to suggest topics (indicated by relevant linguistic variations) such as 'disease dangerous factor', giving rise to large amounts of academic publications that are more likely to be cross-referenced, whereas topics associated with low academic publications such as 'disease dangerous element' and 'disease risk factor' are much less likely to be cited by peer academics.

Table 6.1 summarises the findings in Figs. 6.1, 6.2 and 6.3. In an effort to ascertain whether such patterns hold true for the other conceptual clusters, the distribution and dissemination patterns of other sets of linguistic variations were also analysed and compared based on the corpus-based trend analysis of Chinese research and media publications containing relevant variant translations as keywords in the documents (Figs. 6.4, 6.5, 6.6, 6.7, 6.8, 6.9, 6.10, 6.11, 6.12 and 6.13).

EQUALISATION
Variation 1: 均衡; Variation 2: 平衡; Variation 3: 均衡化
SUSTAINABILITY:
Variation 1: 可持续性; Variation 2: 经济活力; Variation 3: 经济承受能力
(*RIS-ADJUSTED) CAPITATION*
Variation 1: 人头税 (tax per head); Variation 2: 按人头付费 (payment per capita)

Tables 6.1, 6.2, 6.3 and 6.4 show the general patterns of the performance of related linguistic variations within each conceptual cluster. The purpose of this comparison was to find out whether there is any consistent pattern between the three indicators, i.e. Academic Growth Rate (AGR), medium dissemination rate (MDR) and academic disseminate

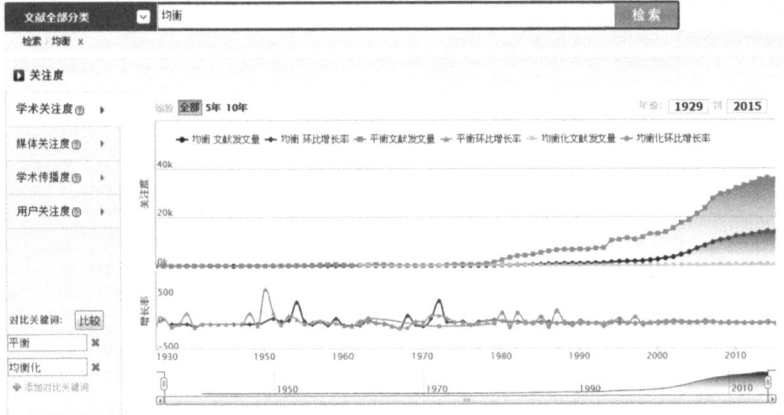

Fig. 6.4 AGR: Distribution patterns of Chinese linguistic variations of '*Equalisation*' in CNKI

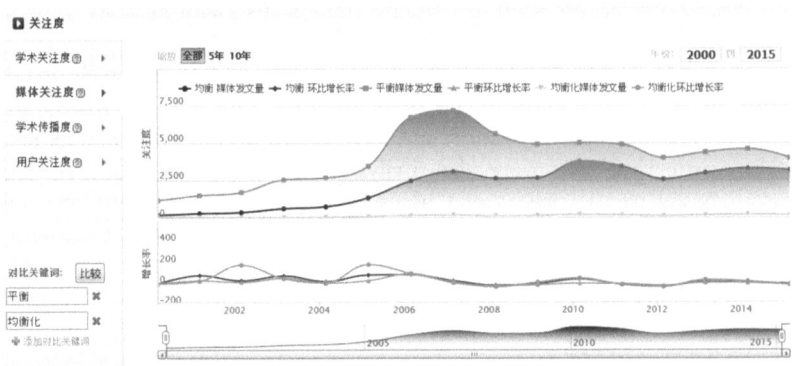

Fig. 6.5 MDR: Distribution patterns of Chinese linguistic variations of '*Equalisation*' in CNKI

rate (ADR). In the detailed analysis of the three linguistic variations of the conceptual cluster 'risk factor', it was found that higher AGR was associated with higher ADR, although there was lack of evidence supporting a similar relationship between ADR and MDR indicating the sectoral nature of academic research and media publications. Such

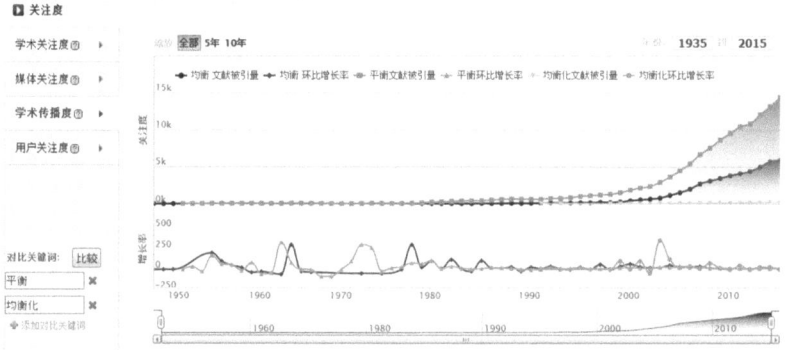

Fig. 6.6 ADR: Distribution patterns of Chinese linguistic variations of '*Equalisation*' in CNKI

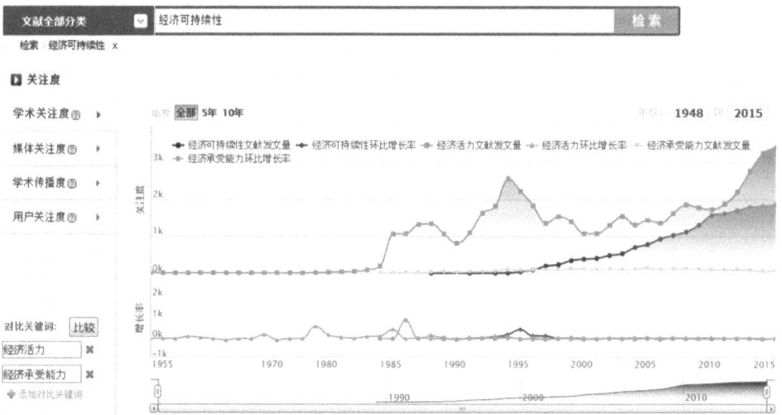

Fig. 6.7 AGR: Distribution patterns of Chinese linguistic variations of '*Sustainability*' in CNKI

observation while holds true for the conceptual cluster 'equalisation', does not seem to fit the data pattern which represent the correlation among linguistic variations belonging to the risk conceptual clusters 'sustainability' and '(risk)-adjusted capitation'.

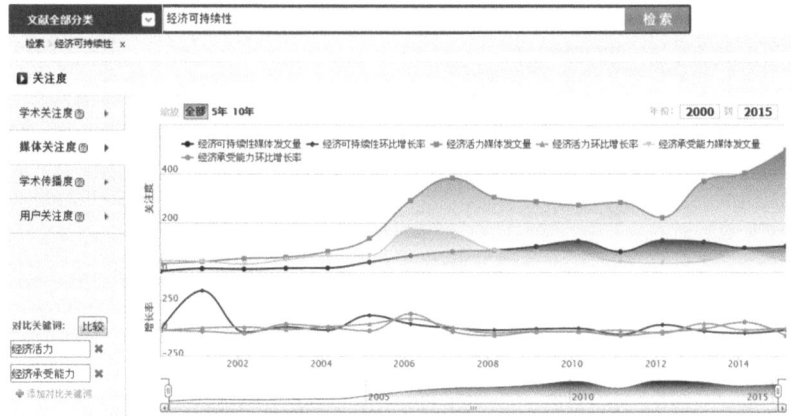

Fig. 6.8 MDR: Distribution patterns of Chinese linguistic variations of '*Sustainability*' in CNKI

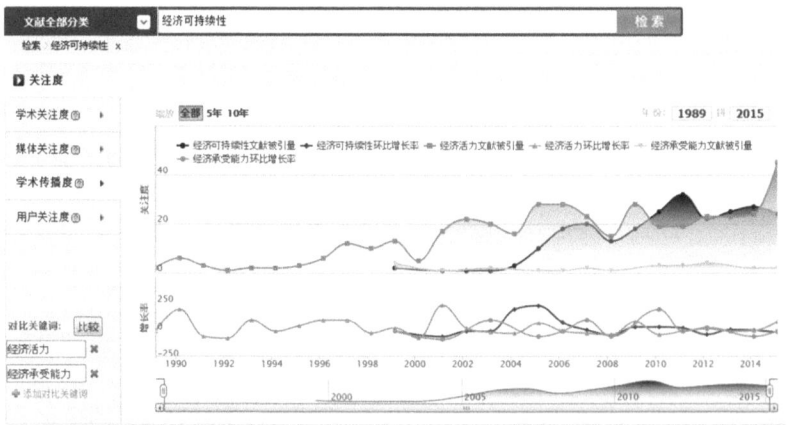

Fig. 6.9 ADR: Distribution patterns of Chinese linguistic variations of '*Sustainability*' in CNKI

The MDR scores for translated terms 3 (Disease Risk Factor) and 6 (Equalisation) are relatively low, whereas the MDR scores for translated terms 9 (Sustainability) and 11 (Payment per Capita) are medium. These suggest that in Chinese printed materials as represented by the CNKI database, arguably the most comprehensive and updated publication

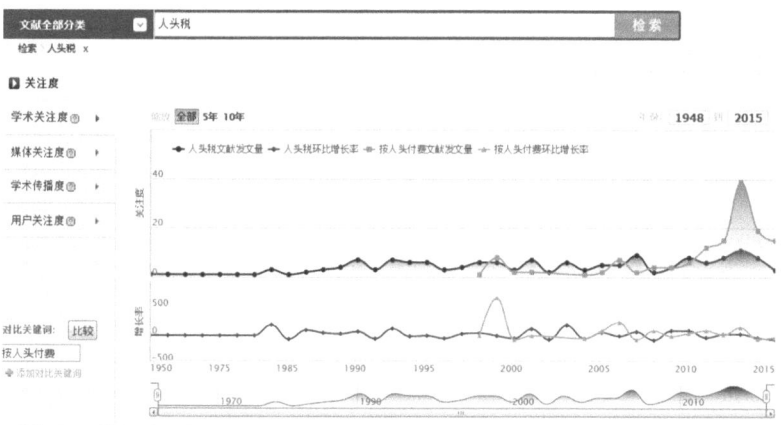

Fig. 6.10 AGR: Distribution patterns of Chinese linguistic variations of 'Capitation' in CNKI

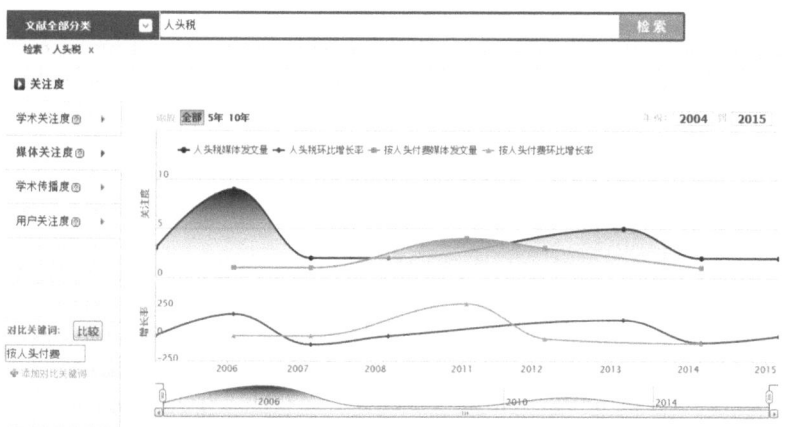

Fig. 6.11 MDR: Distribution patterns of Chinese linguistic variations of 'Capitation' in CNKI

databases in mainland China, there are limited numbers of media reports discussing 'Disease Risk Factor' and (health financial risk) 'Equalisation'. By contrast, there seems to be reasonable amount of public interest and discussion around 'Sustainability' and 'Payment per Capita'.

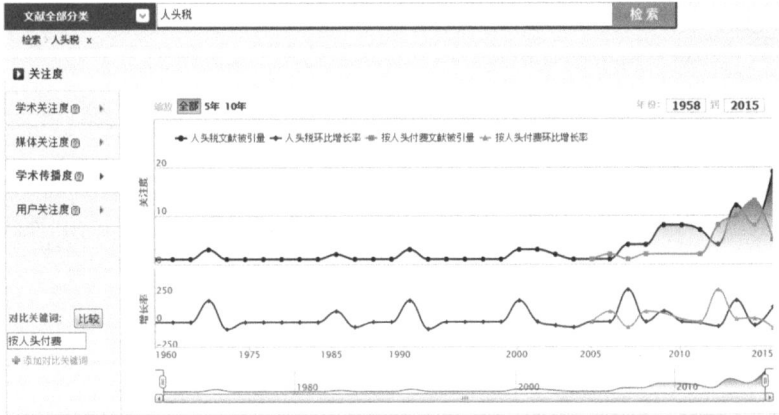

Fig. 6.12 ADR: Distribution patterns of Chinese linguistic variations of 'Capitation' in CNKI

This may be explained by the fact that translated terms 3 'Disease Risk Factor' and 6 (health financial risk) 'Equalisation' are much more complex and specialised expressions and concepts that have not been fully explored in Chinese printed media materials. Differently, translated terms 9 (Sustainability) and 11 (Payment per Capita) have received in-depth media discussion which reflects the public interest on these topics, as well as the relevance and importance of these topics to people's social life and economic activities.

We therefore proceed to test the revised hypothesis that Academic Growth Rate (AGR) instead of being associated with ADR alone, it is related or influenced by the compound impact of the two indicators: Academic Dissemination Rate (ADR) and Media Dissemination Rate (MDR). That is, in the following section, we intend to find out whether dissemination rates in academic and media publications can be used to explain and even to predict the amount and growth level of academic publications on specific health risk topics. This is explored by regression analysis in which we test the relationship between AGR as the dependent variable and ADR and MDR as two explanatory variables. The findings of our analysis will be of important practice use for the development of specialised translation editing and analytical systems.

AGR (4, 5, 6, 9, 3, 7, 2, 11, 10 and 8: numbering of translations along the vertical dendrogram)

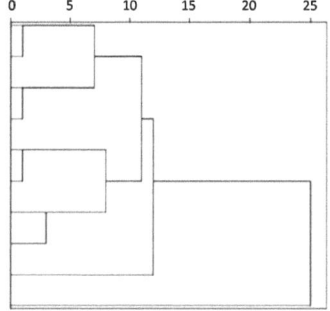

ADR (4, 5, 2, 6, 9, 3, 11, 7, 10, 8, 1: numbering of translations along the vertical dendrogram)

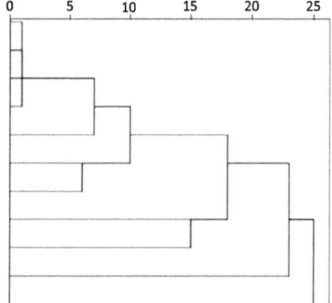

MDR (4, 6, 7, 9, 3, 11, 1, 2, 5, 8, 10: numbering of translations along the vertical dendrogram)

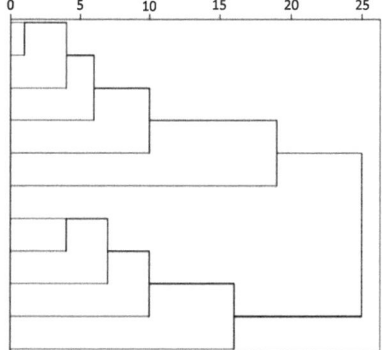

Fig. 6.13 HCA of AGR (*above*), ADR (*middle*) and MDR (*below*). 1 疾病危险因子 (dangerous element); 2 疾病危险因素 (dangerous factor); 3 (T) 疾病风险因素 (risk factor); 4 均衡 (equalise); 5 平衡 (balance); 6 (T) 均衡化 (equalisation); 7 经济活力 (economic dynamics); 8 经济承受能力 (affordability); 9 (T) 可持续性 (sustainability); 10 人头税 (tax per head); 11 (T) 按人头付费 (payment per capita)

Table 6.2 Comparison of variant translations of 'Equalisation' in Chinese research and media publications

Quantitative measures	Balance	Equalise	Equalisation (6)
Academic Growth Rate (AGR)	High	Medium	Low
Academic Dissemination Rate (ADR)	High	Medium	Low
Media Dissemination Rate (MDR)	High	Medium	Low

Table 6.3 Comparison of variant translations of 'Sustainability' in research and media Publications

Quantitative measures	Economic dynamics	Sustainability (9)	Affordability
Academic Growth Rate (AGR)	High	High	Medium
Academic Dissemination Rate (ADR)	High	High	Low
Media Dissemination Rate (MDR)	High	Medium	Medium

Table 6.4 Comparison of variant translations of 'Capitation' in Chinese research and media Publications

Quantitative measures	Tax per head	Payment per capita (11)
Academic Growth Rate (AGR)	Medium	High
Academic Dissemination Rate (ADR)	High	High
Media Dissemination Rate (MDR)	Medium	Medium

6.2 Findings on Inter-indicator Relationships Between ADR, MDR and AGR

6.2.1 Regression Analysis: Exploring Joint Impact of ADR and MDR on AGR

In this study, AGR, ADR and MDR are three indicators of conceptually related translation variations in the target knowledge system. This section intends to test the hypothesis that high ADR and MDR can be used to predict high AGR for health risk terms. We analysed four translations identified in the four conceptual clusters, i.e. 'risk factor', '(risk pooling) equalisation', '(health financial) sustainability' and '(risk-adjusted)

Table 6.5 Summary of regression analysis of Chinese translation of 'Disease Risk Factor'

Model summary

R	R square	Adjusted R square	Std. error of the estimate
0.904	0.816	0.788	24.784

ANOVA

	Sum of squares	Df	Mean square	F	Sig.
Regression	35,492.941	2	17,746.470	28.890	0.000

Table 6.6 Summary of regression analysis of Chinese translation of 'Equalisation'

Model summary

R	R square	Adjusted R square	Std. error of the estimate
0.985	0.971	0.967	27.018

ANOVA

	Sum of squares	Df	Mean square	F	Sig.
Regression	318,335.240	2	159,167.620	218.045	0.000

capitation'. In the regression analysis, we tested the compound impact of the academic and media dissemination rates (ADR and MDR) on the level of the growth of academic knowledge (AGR) on specific health risk topics. The results illustrate the effectiveness of the model by the adjusted R^2 values and F scores and associated significance level in ANOVA test (Analysis of Variation).

Tables 6.5, 6.6, 6.7 and 6.8 show the regression models built for the four translations from the four conceptual clusters. The adjusted R^2 values and F scores obtained in the four models indicate that there is a very strong or strong relationship between the dependent variable, i.e. the amount and level of academic publications on specific health risk topics and the explanatory variables, i.e. the academic dissemination rate and the media dissemination rate of the translated terms under study.

Table 6.7 Summary of regression analysis of Chinese translation of 'Sustainability'

Model summary

R	R square	Adjusted R square	Std. error of the estimate
0.860	0.740	0.700	435.387

ANOVA

	Sum of squares	Df	Mean square	F	Sig.
Regression	7,012,788.177	2	3,506,394.088	18.497	0.000

Table 6.8 Summary of the Chinese translation of 'Capitation'

Model summary

R	R square	Adjusted R square	Std. error of the estimate
0.840	0.706	0.660	5.931

ANOVA

	Sum of squares	Df	Mean square	F	Sig.
Regression	1096.492	2	548.246	15.587	0.000

6.2.2   Clustering Analysis: Exploring Similarities Among Translated Health Risk Terms (ADR and MDR)

Based on the analysis of linguistic variations within each conceptual cluster, this section examines whether translated terminology behave similarly across conceptual clusters when compared to non-translated linguistic expressions. This is achieved by using Hierarchical Cluster Analysis (HCA). HCA is widely used in applied linguistics to develop the hierarchical structure of different samples based on their dissimilarities. The computational modelling of the hierarchical structure of the samples goes through an agglomerative clustering process which starts with the identification of observational variables that are most similar to each other.

Table 6.9 Coding of linguistic variations of health conceptual clusters (translations are indicated by T)

Cluster	Coding	Component linguistic expressions	English translation
I	1	疾病危险因子	Dangerous element
	2	疾病危险因素	Dangerous factor
	3 (T)	疾病风险因素	Risk factor
II	4	均衡	Equalise
	5	平衡	Balance
	6 (T)	均衡化	Equalisation
III	7	经济活力	Economic dynamics
	8	经济承受能力	Affordability
	9 (T)	可持续性	Sustainability
IV	10	人头税	Tax per head
	11 (T)	按人头付费	Payment per capita

At each stage, two observational variables that prove most similar to each other are combined together to form a bottom-level cluster. The procedure continues until similar clusters merge together. HCA is particularly relevant and useful for relatively small datasets like the current study. In this study, average linkage was used to produce a matrix of distance scores indicating the varying levels of dissimilarities among observed variables. Table 6.9 shows the coding of the component linguistic expressions in the four conceptual clusters. Translations are indicated by the letter T next to the coding number.

Despite the relatively small set of corpus data collected and the different temporal distributions (some terms are relatively new, some terms date back to the 1940s) of the variant translations of the four conceptual clusters, interesting and consistent patterns began to emerge in the quantitative analysis. It was found that translated terms shared similar patterns of distribution in Chinese academic and media publications, particularly in terms of the two indicators, ADR and MDR. For example, in Fig. 6.13, ADR3, ADR6, ADR9, ADR11 exhibit some similarities as indicated by their limited level of distance on the graph. ADR3 and ADR11 were emerged to form a cluster.

The level of dissimilarity between ADR3 and ADR11 is indicated by the length of the vertical bar which is roughly at 7 measured by the horizontal axis shown on the top of the graph. The longer the vertical bar, the more dissimilar the two objects under comparison. Similarly, ADR4,

ADR5, ADR2 and ADR6 were merged to form a cluster which went on to annex ADR 9. Lastly, the cluster containing ADR4, ADR5, ADR2, ADR6 and ADR9 was emerged with the cluster containing ADR3 and ADR11. This result detects important similarities in the use of translated terms (3, 6, 9 and 11) in Chinese research and media publication databases, as far as their ADR (academic distribution rate) scores are concerned.

Similarly, in the dendrogram produced for MDR, MDR4 and MDR6 were first emerged due to their shown similarity. This cluster went on to annex ARD7, ADR9 and ADR3 successively and was finally emerged with ADR11 to form the largest cluster in the upper part of the dendrogram. This result indicates that when compared to the ADR scores among translated terms (3, 6, 9 and 11), there are larger dissimilarities between these expressions in terms of their use in Chinese formal media materials. The use of translated term 11 (Payment per Capita) is distinctively different from translated terms 3 (Disease Risk Factor), 6 (Equalisation) and 9 (Sustainability).

This is well illustrated on the dendrogram where the length of the vertical bar which measures the distance between translated term 11 and the rest in the upper cluster is the largest. However, despite the internal differences among translated terms 3, 6, 9 and 11, they have been grouped in one single large cluster in which translated items account for four of the total six observed variables. The upper cluster that they formed stands in clear contrast with the lower cluster on the dendrogram which contains exclusively original Chinese terms.

These findings from the clustering analysis show that on a general level, there are some similarities among translated terms as measured by the two statistical indicators ADR (academic distribution rate) and MDR (media distribution rate). Secondly, the similarities among translated terms are accentuated by the detected differences between translated terms and original Chinese linguistic expressions. This is reflected in the two dendrograms of ADR and MDR. On both figures, translated terms were readily grouped within one large cluster in which translated terms represent the majority: four out of seven of the upper cluster on the ADR graph and four out of six of the upper cluster on the MDR graph. These clusters clearly separate the rest of the observed variables or clusters of observed variables on both of graphs.

Although remain to be further tested with more translation data and materials, such research findings have shed new light on the complexity and subtlety of health policy translation and the subsequent health risk knowledge building in the target culture and society. Using linguistically and culturally embedded expressions, health research institutes can effectively enhance the understanding and dissemination of translated health materials in the academic and media publications in the target language. This in turn can significantly increase the interactive-ness between the source and the target health research and communication systems to close gaps in the understanding and representation of health knowledge; and more importantly, to build much-needed consensus across cultures and societies and develop joint or aligned action plans to tackle global health risks.

CHAPTER 7

Conclusion

Abstract Enhanced public understanding and social awareness of important health research topics such as healthcare financial risks underpins the construction of global consensus and the development of coordinated actions and policy-making across countries to tackle global health risks. This book offered an original empirical study of English to Chinese health translations.

Keywords Health translation strategies · Corpus analysis Knowledge dissemination

In this study, the translations used were official Chinese translations of WHO annual reports and key policy documents. The translation materials were publically available online on the WHO website. The health translation phenomenon investigated was health policy terminological variation. Chinese variant translations of original English expressions were identified and subsequently grouped under various conceptual clusters of health terminologies. The conceptual clusters built facilitated the comparison between variant translations and associated health translation strategies, as well as their interactions which underscored the development of local research and knowledge bodies and enhanced public awareness and understanding of public health risks.

The large-scale corpus analysis of publication trends was feasible with the availability of high-quality research databases such as the Chinese

© The Author(s) 2017
M. Ji, *Translation and Health Risk Knowledge Building in China*,
DOI 10.1007/978-981-10-4681-0_7

Knowledge Resources Integrated Network (or CNKI) in recent years. It enabled the analysis of scientific research and media publication containing key health risk concepts and terms in China since the early twentieth century. The linguistic analysis was based on the study of three indicators generated by the CNKI databases. The corpus analysis demonstrated that high-performance translation variations seemed to be more dynamic and achieved greater social reach in the representation and advancement of translated and introduced public health knowledge. The significance of high-performance translation variants is that they have played and continue to play an instrumental role in informing and transforming the target society.

The outcomes of this study have important theoretical and practical implications. For applied translation studies, it highlighted the needs to adopt translation methods to enhance the intended social impact of translated documents. For empirical translation research, this study illustrated the feasibility and productivity to integrate research methodologies across a range of disciplines for empirical translation studies. In this regard, this study effectively integrated both quantities and qualitative analysis from corpus linguistics, translation studies and contrastive linguistics (Chinese-English) to advance the study of specialised health translations.

Appendix Chinese Translations of Selected Health Financial Risk Terms in WHO Annual Reports

1. *Spreading risk* and subsidising the poor: pooling of resources.
2. 分散投资风险 和资助穷人: 资源的集中共享.
3. Approaches to *spreading risk* and subsidising the poor: country cases.
4. 分散投资风险 和资助穷人的办法: 国家实例.
5. Pooling to *redistribute risk*, and cross-subsidy for greater equity.
6. 共同分散风险, 交叉补助以实现更大公平.
7. South Africa: regulating the private insurance market to increase *risk pooling.*
8. 南非: 调整私营保险市场以增加 风险共担.
9. The challenge facing governments in low-income countries is to reduce the regressive burden of out-of-pocket payment for health by expanding prepayment schemes, which spread *financial risk* and reduce the spectre of catastrophic healthcare expenditures.
10. 在低收入国家中, 政府面临的挑战就是通过扩大预付制度来减少以现金支付卫生服务所带来的逆向负担. 预付制度能够分散 财政风险, 遏制灾难性卫生保健支出的幽灵出现.
11. It connects very well with the other three: reducing the excess mortality of poor and marginalised populations; dealing effectively with the leading *risk factors*; and placing health at the centre of the broader development agenda.
12. 它与其他三个方向紧密关联: 减少贫困和边远人口的过多死亡; 有效地处理主要的危险因素以及将卫生保健置于更为广泛的发展议程的中心.
13. Local and national *risk factors* need to be understood.
14. 必须了解在地方一级和国家一级的风险因素.
15. In the case of revenue pooling, creating as wide a pool as possible is critical to spreading *financial risk* for healthcare, and thus reducing

M. Ji, *Translation and Health Risk Knowledge Building in China*,
DOI 10.1007/978-981-10-4681-0

individual risk and the spectre of impoverishment from health expenditures.

16. 就资金筹集而言， 建立一个尽可能广泛的联合筹集系统对于分散卫生保健的<u>财政风险</u>， 并因此减少个人的风险和降低由于卫生保健支出而贫困化的幽灵，是至关重要的.

17. Achieving greater fairness in financing is only achievable through ***risk pooling***—that is, those who are healthy subsidise those who are sick, and those who are rich subsidise those who are poor.

18. 在资金筹集方面实现更大公正性的唯一可行的方法就是通过<u>风险集资</u>—这就是说，让健康的人资助有病的人，让富有的人资助贫困的人.

19. Strategies need to be designed for expansion of ***risk pooling*** so that progress can be made in such subsidies.

20. 需要设计扩大<u>风险集资</u>的战略， 以便在这种相互补助方面能够取得进展.

21. In middle-income countries the policy route to fair prepaid systems is through strengthening the often substantial mandatory, income-based and ***risk-based*** insurance schemes, again ensuring increased public funding to include the poor.

22. 在中等收入国家中， 建立公平预付制度的政策途径就是加强通常基本上是强制性的， 以收入为基础和<u>以风险为基础的</u>保险制度. 此外就是保证增加公共基金， 以支付穷人加入保险的费用.

23. It matters very much how the system treats people's health needs and how it raises revenues from them, including how much protection it offers them from ***financial risk.***

24. 对如何向他们征税， 包括能向人们提供多少<u>财政风险</u>的保护都有很大影响. 但他还能影响如何满足人们的期望.

25. Concern for the non-health outcomes of the system, for fairly sharing the burden of paying for health so that no one is exposed to great ***financial risk***, and attending to people's wishes and expectations about how they are to be treated, would then be considered luxuries, gaining in importance only as income rises and health improves.

26. 对该体系非健康结果的关切， 例如人们应该平摊费用以不至于使人承担<u>财务上的风险</u>, 满足人们的要求和期望， 被认为是一种奢侈的要求, 应该等到收入增加再满足.

27. And there was nothing like the modern practice of referrals from one level of the system to another, and little protection from ***financial risk*** apart from that offered by charity or by small-scale pooling of contributions among workers in the same occupation.

28. 没有任何像现代医疗的转诊制度那样， 从体系的一个级别到另一个级别， 除了由慈善或小规模同行业工人捐赠的联合机构提供之外， 很少得到<u>资金风险</u>的保障.

29. Reforms to consolidate, extend or merge insurance coverage for greater *risk-sharing* have also occurred in Argentina, Chile, Colombia and Mexico, and a mixture of insurance and out-of-pocket health care has replaced much of the public system throughout the former communist countries.

30. 阿根廷, 智利, 哥伦比亚和墨西哥等国出现的风险分担更强的改革包括: 加强和扩大保险的覆盖面: 而几个前社会主义国家的许多公共体制由一系列保险和现金支付的卫生保健所取代.

31. But because healthcare can be catastrophically costly and the need for it unpredictable, mechanisms for *sharing risk* and providing financial protection are important.

32. 但是, 由于卫生保健可能带来灾难性的花费, 并且对它的需求难以预料, 所以, 建立可以分担风险并提供金融保护的机制就显得非常重要.

33. Mechanisms for *sharing risk* and providing financial protection are more important even than in other cases where people buy insurance, as for physical assets like homes or vehicles, or against the *financial risk* to the family of a breadwinner dying young.

34. 建立分担风险和金融保护的机制, 甚至要比人们因某些原因而购买保险更为重要, 例如为房, 车等物质资产, 或为预防家庭生活支柱英年早逝所带来的风险而购买保险.

35. It is certainly true that financing that is more fairly distributed may contribute to better health, by *reducing the risk* that people who need care do not get it because it would cost too much, or that paying for health care leaves them impoverished and exposed to more health problems.

36. 毫无疑问, 能够被更合理分配的融资, 可以通过降低人们因价格昂贵而无法获得所必需的保健, 或因支付卫生保健费用而导致贫困并面临更多的健康问题的风险, 来促进人们的健康.

37. Greater autonomy can mean that people do not take up an intervention because they perceive the individual benefit to be small or *the risk to be substantial*, and do not value the collective or population benefit.

38. 较大的自主权意味着人们可能因为要保护一己之小利或避免 实质性的风险, 而不采用某项干预措施, 从而不利于集体的利益.

39. One reason why confidentiality seems not to be a problem in these countries may be that there is little private insurance and therefore little *risk of coverage being denied* because a provider reveals some information about a patient.

40. 在这些国家中保密性似乎不成问题的一个原因是, 那里很少有私人保险, 因此几乎没有因泄漏患者的医疗信息而拒保的危险.

41. Fair financing in health systems means that *the risks* each household faces due to the costs of the health system are distributed according to ability to pay rather than to *the risk of illness*.

42. 卫生系统的合理的融资是指 根据支付能力而非<u>疾病的危险</u>来分散每个家庭因支付卫生系统的花费而面临的<u>风险</u>:

43. This situation characterises poorer countries and some middle- and high-income ones, in which at least part of the population is inadequately protected from ***financial risks***.

44. 这种情况存在于大多数较为贫穷的国家和一些中高收入国家中, 其中至少有一部分人得到的<u>金融风险</u>保护不足.

45. The second is solved by assuring that each form of prepayment—through taxes of all kinds, social insurance, or voluntary insurance—is progressive or at least neutral with respect to income, being related to capacity to pay rather than to ***health risk.***

46. 第二个问题则可以通过逐渐扩大所有预付方式的规模—通过各种税收, 社会保险, 或自愿保险—或至少确保收入方面的平均来解决, 与支付能力而非<u>健康风险</u>有关.

47. Arrangements that exempt the destitute from user fees at public facilities, or impose a sliding scale based on socioeconomic characteristics, are attempts to reduce ***the risk associated with out-of-pocket payments.***

48. 免除贫困者在公共设施中的使用费, 或根据人们的社会经济地位按比例减少费用的做法, 可以降低<u>与现金支付有关的风险</u>.

49. And even then, such schemes require relatively high administrative costs to distinguish among users, and typically affect only a small amount of total ***risk-related payments***. (*)

50. 并且尽管如此, 该方法仍需要较高的管理费用来区别用户, 只能代表性地影响全部<u>风险性支付</u>的一小部分. (*)

51. Prepayment that is closely related to ***ex ante risk***, as judged from observable characteristics—***risk-related insurance premiums***, for example, is still preferable to out-of-pocket payment because it is more predictable, and may be justified to the extent that ***the risks*** are under a person's control.

52. 与<u>事先风险</u>密切相关的预付方式, 尽管是根据观察所得的特点来判断的一例如, <u>与风险有关的保险费</u>—仍然优于现金支付的方式, 因为它具有更大的预测能力, 可以在某种程度上证明对<u>风险</u>的控制性.

53. Detailed household surveys show that in Brazil, Bulgaria, Jamaica, Kyrgyzstan, Mexico, Nepal, Nicaragua, Paraguay, Peru, the Russian Federation, Vietnam and Zambia more than 1% of all households had to spend on health half or more of their full monthly capacity to pay, which means that in large countries millions of families are ***at risk of impoverishment.***

54. 详细的家庭调查显示, 在巴西, 保加利亚, 牙买加, 墨西哥, 尼泊尔, 尼加拉瓜, 巴拉圭, 秘鲁, 俄联邦, 越南和赞比亚等国, 有1%的家庭将每月花销的一半或一半以上用于健康, 这意味着在较大的国家内, 有成百万的家庭<u>处于贫困的危险中</u>.

55. Generally, high values of equality are associated with predominantly prepaid financing, but Brazil shows extreme inequality despite a high share of prepayment, because of the great inequality in incomes and the large number of families _**at risk of impoverishment**_.

56. 一般来说，预付资金占优势的国家公平指数较高，但是尽管巴西的预付比例较高，但却表现出极度的不公平性，原因在于收入悬殊及有大量的家庭处于贫困的危险中.

57. That means that there is no need to estimate the "coverage" of the population by different _**risk-sharing schemes.**_ (*)

58. 这意味着没有必要根据不同风险承担方案估计人口的"保险范围". (*)

59. To make matters more complicated, a given intervention may be effective against more than one disease or cause, because it works on a _**common risk factor**_ or symptom. (*)

60. 使问题更加复杂化的是，某一特定的干预会作用于一个以上的疾病或病因，因为其作用于一个普遍的危险因子或症状. (*)

61. Family planning, prenatal and delivery care, clean and safe delivery by trained birth attendant, postpartum care, and essential obstetric care for _**high-risk pregnancies**_ and complications.

62. 计划生育，产前与分娩保健，由经过培训的接生人员进行干预,产后保健，以及针对高危妊娠及其综合征的基础产科保健.

63. A health system ought to protect people from _**financial risk**_, to be consistent with the goal of fair financial contribution.

64. 一个卫生体制就应该保护人们避免财政危险，而达到公平享受资金分配的目标.

65. Too narrow an approach also ignores the important role that the public sector should be playing in protecting the poor and addressing insurance market failure—the tendency of insurance to exclude precisely those people who need it most, because they are _**at greater than usual risk of ill-health**_. (*)

66. 某种太有限的途径，也忽略了公共部门应该起保护穷人和强调保险市场失败的重要角色，保险的趋势是精确地除外那些最需要它的人们，因为他们 比通常的疾病与健康危险比率都高. (*)

67. When protection from catastrophic cost is the overriding consideration and prepayment can _**protect against that risk.**_

68. 当对灾难性成本的保护被置之不理或预付资金可以保护免受此灾难时.

69. Major progress has been made recently in understanding global health and disease patterns, including analysis of _**risk factors**_ which influence several diseases at once.

70. 最近，人们已经在了解全球卫生和疾病形式方面获得了很大的进展，这包括对能够立即影响严重疾病危险因子的分析.

71. The most significant of such _**risk factors**_ are malnutrition in children, and poor water and sanitation practices.

72. 这些<u>危险因子</u>最重要的是儿童营养不良以及缺水和<u>卫生</u>问题.

73. Other major ***risk factors*** include unsafe sex, alcohol, indoor pollution, tobacco, occupational hazards, hypertension and physical inactivity.

74. 其他主要<u>危险因子</u>包括不安全的性活动，酒精，室内污染，烟草，职业危害，高血压和物理性静止.

75. The public health services in a given country should attempt to deal with such ***preventable risk factors***, taking account of local contexts. (*)

76. 某一确定国家的公共卫生服务应该力图解决这些<u>预防性危险因子</u>，也包括当地的各种因素. (*)

77. Public health activities will therefore vary, depending on local ***risk factors*** and diseases conditions.

78. 根据当地<u>危险因子</u>和疾病条件的不同，公共卫生活动也将因此变化.

79. Although there are good data on national ***patterns of risk*** and disease today, few countries break this information down sub-nationally by income level, sex or vulnerable groups, such as the handicapped, minority ethnic populations, and the frail elderly. (*)

80. 尽管今天我们已经有了各国 <u>危险因子和疾病形式</u> 的良好资料，但很少有国家根据以下各项在亚国家水平上进行分解，这些项目包括：收入水平，性别或易感人群，例如残疾，少数民族人群以及虚弱的老人等. (*)

81. A key recommendation for policy-makers is to collect and combine data on ***risk factors,*** health conditions and interventions with data from household and facilities surveys, focus groups and other qualitative methods, and academic studies, since global and national aggregate data may not reflect local needs.

82. 一个对政策制订者的重要建议就是收集和综合有关<u>危险因子</u>，卫生状况以及来自各户和机构调查，目标人群和其他定性方法，学术研究中的资料，因为全球各个国家的集合性资料可能不能反映地方的需求.

83. First, there should be an ongoing detailed assessment of ***underlying risk factors***, disease burden and utilisation patterns of the target populations. (*)

84. 首先，应该有一个正在进行且详细的评估系统，以分析 <u>危险因子</u>，疾病负担以及目标人群的使用形式. (*)

85. This is relatively common in private insurance, either by explicit exclusion of services or by ***risk selection*** of potential clients so as to reduce the likelihood of those services.

86. 这在私人保险中相当普遍，无论是通过拨款除外的服务方式，还是对潜在客户进行<u>危险选择</u>以减少这些服务的可能性的方式.

87. But it maximises people's exposure to ***financial risk*** if the intervention can be had by paying out of pocket or to catastrophic health losses, if the service is simply not available at all.

88. 但如果支付现金来获得干预，   这会使人们最大限度地暴露在<u>财政危险</u>的境遇中， 或者如果只是简单地丝毫没有获得服务， 则可能导致健康损失的灭顶之灾.

89. But some priorities can nonetheless be enforced through regulation, as for example by requiring all private insurance policies to include a package of essential services or by limiting the degree to which private providers or insurers can select patients or clients ***on the basis of risk.*** (*)

90. 但是尽管如此， 一些优点也可以通过法规来得到加强， 例如要求所有的私人保险政策都包括一个基础服务包， 或者限制私人提供者和保险人用来选择病人或客户的<u>危险基线的程度</u>. (*)

91. The growing awareness of the structural nature of problems in hierarchical service delivery systems has led policy-makers in many countries to examine the incentive environment of organisations and alter the distribution of decision-making control, revenue rights, and ***financial risk*** among the different participants, as analysed in The world health report 1999.

92. 在等级性服务体制中对于结构特性的不断认识，   已经使得许多国家的政策制定者在检查组织奖励环境， 并开始改变决策控制， 收入权利和<u>财政风险</u>在不同参与者之间的分布. 参见《1999年世界卫生报告》.

93. Where the share of total revenues earned through markets is significant, organisations are ***at financial risk*** because of the unrecoverable costs associated with requirements for which no funds are provided, such as care for the poor or very sick.

94. 通过市场挣取的总收入的份额是很重要的，   组织仍然<u>面临财政危险</u>，这是由于有与没有资金支持的一些要求相关的无给付成本的存在， 例如对穷人和严重疾病患者的治疗.

95. ***Financial risk*** remains limited. Actual degree of market exposure may be greater than intended when user fees are significant.

96. <u>财政风险</u>保持在有限的程度. 市场暴露的实际程度要比预期的大， 这是当使用者费用有意义的时候.

97. As organisational units like hospitals or clinics become more autonomous, the service delivery system is ***at risk of becoming fragmented***.

98. 当像医院或诊所这样的组织单位变得更加自主时， 服务提供系统也 <u>面临着被肢解的危险</u>.

99. New investment choices must be made carefully to reduce the ***risk of future imbalances***, and the existing mix of inputs needs to be monitored on a regular basis.

100. 新的投资选择必须谨慎进行， 以减少<u>未来不平衡的风险</u>， 并使现存投资需求的混合在规范的基础上得到监督.

101. In order to ensure fairness and ***financial risk protection,*** there should be a high level of prepayment; risk should be spread (through

cross-subsidies from low to high health risk); the poor should be subsidised (through cross-subsidies from high to low income).

102. 为了确保公正性和投资风险防护, 应当建立高水平的预付金, 投资风险应当通过对由低健康危险因素到高健康危险因素的交叉资助 予以分散, 穷人应当通过对由高收入者到低收入者进行的交叉资助得到资助;

103. Health systems have various ways of collecting revenue, such as general taxation, mandated social health insurance contributions (usually salary-related and almost never risk-related), voluntary private health insurance contributions (usually *risk-related*), out-of-pocket payment and donations.

104. 卫生系统有许多不同的方式得到收入, 如一般税, 强制性社会健康保险费用收入(常常是与工资相关的, 并且几乎没有风险), 自愿性个人健康保险费用收入(常常有风险), 医疗支付费用以及捐赠款项.

105. Pooling is the accumulation and management of revenues in such a way as to ensure that the *risk of having to pay* for healthcare is borne by all the members of the pool and not by each contributor individually.

106. 集资是指为保证将卫生保健付费的风险由所有集资者来承担, 而非由其中的某一个体来承担的一种对所得收入进行积累和管理的方法.

107. Its main purpose is to share the *financial risk* associated with health interventions for which the need is uncertain.

108. 其主要目的就是要使与各种需求不明确的卫生干预相关的财务风险得到分散.

109. The way policy-makers organise public financing or influence private financing will affect four key determinants of health system financing performance: the level of prepayment; the *degree of spreading of risk*; the extent to which the poor are subsidised; and strategic purchasing.

110. 政策制订者组织公共融资或影响私人融资的方法将影响卫生系统融资性能的四个决定因素: 即预先支付的水平, 风险的分散程度, 穷人受到资助的程度以及有计划性的购买.

111. Fairness of *financial risk protection* requires the highest possible degree of separation between contributions and utilisation.

112. 风险防护的合理性需要出资与用资两者最大可能地得到分离.

113. In addition to affording protection against having to pay out of pocket and, as a result, facing barriers to access, prepayment makes it possible to spread the *financial risk* among members of a pool, as discussed later in the chapter.

114. 除了防止必须由个人自己来承担费用进而使可以享受卫生服务的人的范围受到限制以外, 预先支付还使得财政风险在参与融资者中得到分散成为可能, 本章后面将对这种情况予以讨论.

115. Individual out-of-pocket financing does not allow the risk to be shared in that way.

116. 个人现金支付的方式不允许投资风险以上述的方式得到分散.

117. In middle-income countries, with more formal economies, strategies to increase prepayment as well as pooling arrangements include strengthening and expanding mandatory salary-based or ***risk-based contribution systems***, as well as increasing the share of public financing, particularly for the poor.

118. 在中等收入的国家，经济体制相比较为正规完善，增加预先支付以及融资的规划包括加强和推广强制性基于工资或<u>基于风险的出资系统</u>，以及增加公共融资的比重(尤其对穷人).

119. Pooling is the main way to ***spread risks*** among participants.

120. 集资是参与者 <u>分散风险</u> 的主要形式.

121. People with ***a high risk of having to use services***, such as the sick and the elderly, would be denied access because they could not save enough from their income.

122. 那些<u>卫生服务的高需求人群</u>(如病人或者老年人)将可能由于不能从他们的收入中拿出足够的钱存入医疗存款账户而失去得到卫生服务的权利.

123. On the other hand, the healthy and the young, whose risk is usually low, might prepay for a long time without needing the services for which they had saved.

124. 另一方面，健康人以及年轻人对需要卫生服务的风险较低，他们可能会将他们的钱预先支付了很长时间，但并不需要他们预先支付的卫生服务.

125. Thus, systems as well as people benefit from mechanisms that not only increase the degree of prepayment for health services, but also spread the ***financial risk*** among their members.

126. 因此，卫生服务预先支付程度增加的同时，将 <u>融资风险</u> 分散到所有参与者的这一机制，将使得卫生系统以及公众受益.

127. As a result of large pools, society takes advantage of economies of scale, the law of large numbers, and ***cross-subsidies from low-risk to high-risk individuals***. (*)

128. 作为大型集资的一个结果，社会得益于规模(即大型的)经济 以及 <u>由高风险人群向低风险人群进行的交叉资助</u>. (*)

129. Pooling by itself allows for equalisation of contributions among members of the pool regardless of their ***financial risk associated with service utilisation***. But it also allows the low-risk poor to subsidise the high-risk rich.

130. 集资本身容许在不考虑每个参与者 <u>使用卫生服务的出资风险</u> 的前提下，将出资份额平均分摊到集资参与者的每个人头上，且其也容许低风险的穷人去资助高风险的富人.

131. Therefore, health financing, in addition to ensuring ***cross-subsidies from low to high risk*** (which will happen in any pool, unless ***contributions***

are risk-related), should also ensure that such subsidies are not regressive.

132. 因此，卫生融资应确保其 交叉资助的方向是由低风险朝向高风险（对于一切集资，除非 出资是与风险相关的），并且应确保这种交叉资助不能反向运作.

133. Health systems throughout the world attempt to *spread risk* and subsidise the poor through various combinations of organisational and technical arrangements.

134. 全世界的卫生系统都努力 分散投资风险 并通过不同组合的组织及技术安排来资助穷人.

135. Both *risk- and income-related cross-subsidies* could occur among the members of the same pool, for example in single pool systems such as the Costa Rican social security organisation and the national health service in the UK, or via government subsidies to a single or multiple pool arrangement.

136. 风险相关的交叉资助和收入相关的交叉资助 可以存在于同一集资体的参与者之中，如哥斯达黎加的社会保障组织以及英国的国家卫生服务之类的单一集资系统，或者也可以通过政府对单一或多个集资安排的资助基金.

137. In practice, in the majority of health systems, *risk and income cross-subsidisation* occurs via a combination of two approaches: pooling and government subsidy.

138. 实际上在大多数的卫生系统中，风险相关的交叉资助以及收入相关的交叉资助 通过两种手段的结合出现，这两种手段就是集资和政府基金.

139. Cross-subsidisation can also occur among members of different pools (in a multiple pool system) via explicit *risk and income equalisation mechanisms*, such as those being used in the social security systems of Argentina, Colombia and the Netherlands. (*)

140. 对于含多个集资体的系统，交叉资助也可以通过明确的风险公平性及收入公平性机制 出现于不同集资体中的集资参与者之间，如阿根廷，哥伦比亚，荷兰等国家所实行的就是这样的机制. (*)

141. In these countries, the existence of multiple pools allows members of pools to have different *risk and income profiles*.

142. 在这些国家中，多个集资体的存在使得集资的参与者们可以有着不同的风险背景及收入背景.

143. Without some compensatory mechanisms, such arrangements would offer incentives for pooling organisations to *select low risks*, and to exclude the poor and the sick. (*)

144. 如果没有补偿机制，这样的安排会促使集资资助去选择更低的投资风险，并且排斥穷人和生病的人. (*)

145. Even under single-pool organisations, decentralisation, unless accompanied by equalisation mechanisms for resource allocation, may result in significant risk and income differences among decentralised regions.

146. 即使是单一的集资组织，除非伴有公平的资源分配机制，否则分散化可能在分散的区域之间导致显著的风险和收入的差异.

147. Table 5.2 shows four country examples of different arrangements for **_spreading risk_** and subsidising the poor.

148. 表5.2显示了四个国家的分散投资风险及资助穷人的不同安排的实例.

149. Figure 5.1 Pooling to **_redistribute risk_**, and cross-subsidy for greater equity

150. 表5.1集资 分散风险，交叉资助以实现更大公平.

151. Table 5.2 Approaches to **_spreading risk_** and subsidising the poor: country cases

152. 表5.2 风险分散 以及资助穷人的手段: 国家举例.

153. Intra-pool via non-risk-related contribution and inter-pool via a **_central risk equalisation fund_**.

154. 非风险相关的出资的内部集资以及 集中风险公平性基金.

155. The argument for large pools is therefore not an argument for single pools when multiple pools can exist without fragmentation, and when their size and financing mechanisms allow for adequate **_spreading of risk_** and subsidisation of the poor.

156. 因此，我们所提倡的大型化集资体并非是当多个集资体能够在无分散化的情况下存在，并且其规模及融资体制能够充分地使得投资风险得到分散及穷人得到资助的时候去提倡单一的集资体.

157. Introducing regulations such as community rating (**_adjusting for the average risk of a group_**), portable employment-based pooling (insurance that a worker keeps when changing jobs) and equal minimum benefit packages (access to the same services in all pools), in addition to protecting members of the pools, may pave the way for larger pooling in the future.

158. 引入各种调节机制，如社区评估(根据某一人群的平均危险因素作出调节)，可携带的基于工作的集资(当工作者更换工作时可以继续保持的保险)，以及公平性最低限度利益组合包(集资体内的所有参与者都享有同等的卫生服务)，就可以在为集资体的参与者提供保障的同时为未来的大型化的集资铺平道路.

159. Mandatory participation (that is, all eligible members must join the pooling organisation) significantly reduces the scope of selection behaviour but does not totally eliminate the incentives associated with it, particularly under **_non-risk-related contribution schemes_**.

160. 强制性参与(即所有适合的个体都必须加入该集资组织)显著地减少了选择行为的范围，但是其并未完全消除与选择行为有关的诱因，尤其对于那些非风险相关的出资方案 就更是如此.

161. It is particularly a problem for competition under ***non-risk-related contribution schemes***. Either pooling organisations will try to pick the lowest risk consumers (risk selection), who will contribute but not cause expense, or the highest risk consumers will seek coverage more actively than the rest of the population (adverse selection).

162. 对于 非风险相关的出资方案 情况下的竞争, 其更加成为一个严重的问题. 集资组织要么会努力选择低风险的消费者, 即那些出资却不导致花费的个体(即风险选择), 要么会选择高风险的消费者, 即那些比在同一人群内的其他个体更加积极地寻求保障的个体(即反向选择).

163. Pooling competition then becomes a battle for information between consumers (who usually know more about their own risk of requiring health interventions) and the pooling organisation (which needs to know more about ***consumers' risks*** to ensure long term financial sustainability).

164. 这样一来, 集资竞争就成为一种在消费者(他们通常更了解自身对各种卫生干预需求的风险)与集资组织(它们需要更多地了解消费者的各种卫生干预需求的风险, 用以确保长期的财务支持)之间的信息战.

165. If instead ***risk selection*** predominates, as is most likely when there is weak regulation of pooling competition, the poor and the sick will be excluded.

166. 如果 风险选择 占主要地位(当对于集资竞争的调节比较薄弱时最经常出现), 穷人以及患病者将受到排斥.

167. Regulation may cover such aspects as mandatory participation, ***non-risk-related contributions*** or community rating (the same price for a group of members sharing the same geographical area or the same workplace), and prohibition of underwriting (requesting additional information regarding health risks).

168. 调节包括了诸多方面, 如强制性参与, 非风险相关的出资 或社区评估(同一地区内或同一工作地点的所有参与者享有同等的价格), 禁止保险包销(需要有关卫生服务需求风险的额外信息)等等.

169. Financial incentives may include ***risk compensation mechanisms*** and subsidies for the poor to join a pool.

170. 财政鼓励可以包括 风险补偿机制 以及为使穷人加入某个集资体而设的基金.

171. There are, however, a few instances in the world where attempts have been made to separate the functions and allocate resources from a pooling organisation to multiple purchasers through ***risk-adjusted capitation***.

172. 但是, 世界上也有一些少数的例子做出努力将这两项功能分离并将资金由集资组织通过 风险调整的人头税分配给多个购买方.

173. Such units make it easier for the purchaser and the provider to agree on a payment mechanism in which the provider *shares the risk* with the purchaser.

174. 这样的购买单位使得卫生服务措施的提供方与卫生服务措施的购买方更容易在它们双方共同　承担风险(即卫生服务措施的提供方也要对由相对固定数量资金购买的一套范围齐全的卫生干预措施负部分责任)的支付机制问题上达成协议.

175. The spectrum of *risk sharing*, from all the risk borne by the purchaser to all of it transferred to providers, is discussed in the world health report 1999.

176. 风险分担的各种问题,　从所有风险由卫生服务措施的购买方产生到所有风险都转移到卫生服务措施的提供方都在《1999年世界卫生报告》中有所讨论.

177. If the purchasing unit is too small, the purchaser will have difficulty in agreeing on a *risk sharing payment mechanism,* because of the potential fragmentation of the pool, and will have to resort to traditional input purchasing or fee-for-service.

178. 如果购买单位规模过小,　则卫生服务措施的购买方将由于集资体潜在的分散化而难于在　风险分担支付机制上达成协议,　并且将不得不采取传统的投入购买力方式,　或称收费服务的购买方式.

179. Such a situation will force the purchaser to focus on short-term isolated interventions, as the absence of a *risk sharing agreement* will make it difficult to conclude a long-term contract for interventions for groups of the population.

180. 不能达成　风险分担协议　将使得人群卫生干预措施的长期合同难于签订,　进而将迫使卫生服务措施的购买方专注于短期的单独分离的卫生干预措施.

181. It has been used in the UK National Health Service with regard to general practitioners and later played a more important role in *sharing risk* with the introduction of general practitioner fundholding, allowing surpluses to be invested in the fundholder's practice.

182. 其已被对于全科医生的英国国家卫生服务所采用,　并在引入全科医生资金持有方式之后在　风险分担　方面扮演了更加重要的角色,　允许把多余的资金投入资金持有者的运作之中.

183. When *risk-sharing payment mechanisms* are used, depending on the specific terms of the payment mechanism, part of the pooling function of *spreading risk* among members of the pool may be performed by the provider.

184. 当　风险分担的支付机制　被应用时,　依照支付机制的特定术语,　部分将　风险分担　至所有集资参与者的集资的功能,　可以由卫生干预措施的提供方来完成.

185. There is thus a ***risk of fragmenting the pool*** if the provider groups are too small.

186. 由此可知, 如果这些卫生干预措施提供方过于小型化, 那么将产生 集资分散的风险.

187. In summary, purchasers need to move from supply-side payment to demand-side provider payment mechanisms, from implicit to explicit contracting, and from fee-for-service to some form of ***risk sharing payment mechanisms.***

188. 总而言之, 卫生干预措施的购买方需要从供应方支付转向要求附带的供应方支付机制, 从不明确性转向明确性的签约方式, 以及从收费服务型转向风险分担型的支付机制.

189. Contracting, shifting to demand side payment, and introducing risk sharing provider payment mechanisms require a high level of technical, organisational and institutional capacity, as well as significant political leverage because of the likely resistance of providers to ***bearing more risk*** and being held more accountable, particularly in the public sector.

190. 转向要求附带支付的签约以及引入分散分担的卫生干预措施提供方的支付机制, 需要高水平的技术, 组织以及机构能力, 并且因卫生干预措施提供方(尤其是公立部门)可能产生的对 承担过大风险 以及负担过多责任的抵触, 而需要伴有相当的政策倾斜.

191. Some of the most important factors affecting the performance of health financing organisations and, through it, the ***financial risk protection*** provided by the health system are discussed below.

192. 下面将讨论影响卫生融资组织的有效性的一些最重要的因素, 以及进一步的卫生系统所提供的 财政风险保护 等问题.

193. Private health insurance fund (regulated or unregulated), mostly relying on voluntary contributions (premiums), which may be ***risk-related*** but are usually not income-related, and are often contracted by an employer for all a firm's employees.

194. 私人卫生保险基金(受或不受调节的), 大多依靠自愿出资(保险费), 可能是风险相关 的, 但通常不是收入相关的, 常常由雇主为该公司的所有员工签约.

195. Providers can play a role as pooling organisations under a ***non-risk-adjusted capitation payment*** mechanism, as discussed above.

196. 如上所述, 在 非风险调整人头税的支付机制中, 卫生干预措施的提供方可以扮演如同集资组织的角色.

197. This is particularly evident in comparing private ***risk-related health insurance*** with social security. Social security organisations spread risk among the whole pool through ***non-risk-related contributions***. All members of the pool pay a proportion of their salary, regardless of their risk. In contrast, voluntary private health insurance contributions

charge the same premium only for the members of a similar risk category in the pool (such as the same sex, age and place of residence).

198. 这一点在对比私人 风险相关的卫生保险 与社会保障的时候尤为明显. 社会保障组织通过 非风险相关的出资 将风险分散到整个集资体. 无论他们的风险如何, 集资体的所有参与者都付出他们工资的一部分. 相反地, 自愿性的私人卫生保险的出资仅对于集资体内相似风险级别的成员(如相同性别, 年龄, 居住地点的成员)才收取相同水平的保险费.

199. There are multiple categories in private health insurance, and members are charged according to the ***risk category*** to which they belong. The social security and risk-related private insurance approaches are contradictory, and their coexistence creates different incentives for consumers.

200. 私人卫生保险有着多个风险级别, 每个成员依照他或她所属的级别交纳费用. 社会保障方式以及风险相关的私人保险方式两者是相互对立的, 它们的共存为消费者提供了不同的鼓励.

201. All consumers whose ***risk category*** is such that private insurance would charge them less than the amount that they would have to pay under social insurance have the incentive to avoid contributing to social insurance and use private insurance if they are allowed to.

202. 如果允许的话, 所有那些 风险级别 使得他们的私人保险费用低于他们所要支付的社会保险费用的那些消费者, 将受到鼓励去避免社会保险而去选择私人保险.

203. High-risk people, however, have the incentive to contribute to social security, loading it with ***high-risk members*** and increasing the per capita cost of services for members of the pool.

204. 但是, 高卫生干预措施需求风险者受到参与社会保障体系的鼓励, 使得后者充满了 高风险的成员, 从而增加了集资体成员的每人平均的卫生服务成本.

205. Some health systems with multiple social security organisations have introduced central collecting agencies in charge of ***risk equalisation*** among pools (as in Colombia, Germany and the Netherlands).

206. 一些有着多个社会保障组织的卫生系统(如哥伦比亚, 德国及荷兰)引入了中央收取机构来负责各个集资体之间的风险公平化.

207. In contrast with FONASA which charges all members the same 7% payroll tax irrespective of the risk, ISAPREs are allowed to adjust the contribution (with the 7% payroll tax as a minimum contribution) and the benefit package to ***the risk of*** the principal and his or her family.

208. 国家卫生基金不考虑卫生干预措施的需求风险而向所有的参与者都收取同样的7%的工资税, 而私人卫生保险组织则按照主要委托人及其家庭的卫生干预措施的需求风险来相应地调整其利益组合包以及其出资水平(最低按其工资的7%来出资).

209. Conceptual analysis of the necessity and feasibility of introducing mechanisms for *__risk adjustment__* and portability of public 20 subsidies in the health insurance system of Chile.

210. 智利医疗体系引入风险调节机制 的必要性与可行性以及公众补助可移植性的概念分析.

211. While FONASA is based on salary-related contributions with no exclusions, ISAPREs in practice are based on *__risk-related contributions__*.

212. 国家卫生基金没有例外地依靠基于工资的出资, 而私人卫生保险组织则实际上依靠 风险相关的出资.

213. ISAPREs focused on the richest, and *__risk-selected__* the healthiest.

214. 私人卫生保险组织专注于最富有的人群以及 依照低风险原则 挑选的最健康的人群.

215. Only recently has it been possible to introduce regulation to reduce *__risk selection.__*

216. 直到最近才有了引入减少风险选择 的调节机制的可能.

217. Segmentation has determined that while more than 9% of the total Chilean population is older than 60 years of age(generally *__the highest risk group__* in the population), that population group represents only about 3% of ISAPRE beneficiaries.

218. 市场的分散化决定了在60岁以上人口(一般来说是人口中的 最高风险因素人群)占智利总人口9%的同时, 这类人群仅占到私人卫生保险组织受益人的3%.

219. While ministries of health or finance can respond to unfunded mandates by adjusting the quality or opportunity of interventions or even generating budget deficits, private insurance funds might respond by excluding members who are *__at a high risk of__* requiring the services required by the unfunded mandates.

220. 卫生部或财政部对于无注资的指令的反应可以是调整卫生干预措施的质量及获取机会, 或甚至是用产生预算赤字的方式, 而私人保险基金的反应就可能是排除那部分对于那些种无注资指令中要求的卫生干预措施有着高需求风险的参与者.

221. To avoid negative equity consequences, particularly under increasing autonomy, regulatory and financial incentives (e.g. *__risk compensation mechanisms__*) are necessary to protect the sick and the poor.

222. 为了避免这些尤其是在自主水平逐渐增加的情况下出现的对公平性的负面影响, 需要有调节以及财政鼓励措施(如风险补偿机制)来保护穷人以及生病的人.

223. *__Risk selection__* is almost certain, taking high-income low-risk consumers out of the public pools and worsening the financial situation of the latter.

224. 从公共的集资体中选择高收入, 低卫生干预措施需求风险的消费者并使公共集资体的财政处境恶化的风险选择 将几乎是肯定的.

225. Out-of-pocket payment is usually the most regressive way to pay for health, and the way that most exposes people to catastrophic *financial risk.*

226. 现金支付通常是卫生干预措施支付方法中最落后的, 也是最会将人们暴露于灾难性的<u>财政风险</u>的支付方式.

227. But even if nearly any form of prepayment is preferable, on these grounds, to out-of-pocket spending, it also matters greatly how the revenues are combined so as to share risks: how many pools there are, how large they are, whether inclusion is voluntary or mandatory, whether exclusion is allowed, what degree and kind of competition exists among pools, and whether, in the case of competing pools, there are mechanisms to compensate for *differences in risk and in capacity to pay.*

228. 即使几乎任何方式的预先支付在这种情况下都比现金支付要强, 但是如何去组合这些所得收入从而将风险分散还是十分重要的. 其包括共有多少个集资体存在, 这些集资体的规模有多大, 这些集资体的参与是自愿的还是强制性的, 是否允许这些集资体对于一些进行排除, 集资体之间存在何种程度及种类的竞争, 以及对于竞争性的集资体来说是否存在<u>风险及支付能力差异</u>的补偿机制.

229. All these features affect the fairness of the system, but they also help determine how efficiently it operates. The argument in favour of a single pool or a small number of pools of adequate size, and against fragmentation, concerns the financial viability of pools, the administrative costs of insurance, the balance between the economies of scale and (when there is little or no competition) *the risks of capture and unresponsiveness,* and the limitation of *risk selection* (which is a matter of efficiency as well as equity).

230. 所有这些问题都影响到该系统的公平性, 但是它们也帮助确定了该系统的有效率性. 赞成单独集资体或少量足够规模的集资体, 反对分散化的观点涉及到一些问题, 如各个集资体的财政生存, 卫生保险的行政管理费用, 规模经济与(当少无或无竞争时的)<u>决策受制及无反应性的风险</u> 之间的平衡, 以及 <u>风险选择</u> 的限制(其既是效率问题, 又是公平性问题).

231. South Africa has recently changed earlier regulations governing medical schemes to reduce *risk selection* and increase *risk pooling.*

232. 最近南非修改了管理医疗方案的早期法规, 以减少<u>风险选择</u> 和增加<u>风险共保</u>.

233. Chile has been unable to establish explicit contractual obligations for private insurers or prohibit *risk selection* by these private companies, due to the political influence of insurers and their clients.

234. 由于保险公司及其委托人的政治影响, 智利已不能给私立保险公司制定明确的合同义务, 或不能阻止这些私营保险公司的<u>风险选择</u>.

235. South Africa: regulating the private insurance market to increase *risk pooling.*

236. 南非：控制私营保险市场以增加 风险共担.

237. The private sector responded to this by limiting benefits, increasing co-payments and accelerating the exclusion of *high-risk members* from cover, thereby heightening the problem of inequality.

238. 私立部门对通货膨胀做出以下反应：限定给付，增加附加付费，加速从参保者中排除高风险会员，从而加剧了不平等.

239. The new government's response to these challenges was to enact new legislation for medical schemes to offer a minimum benefits package and increased *risk pooling.*

240. 新政府对这些挑战的反应是颁布新的医疗方案法规，提供一个最小福利范围，增加 风险共保.

241. *Risk* or age *rating* is prohibited.

242. 禁止 风险定费 或年龄定费.

243. Increased *risk pooling.*

244. 增加 风险共保.

245. Caps on the permissible contributions and accumulations through individual medical savings accounts will ensure that a greater proportion of contributions flows into the common *risk pool.*

246. 对允许分摊额和通过个人医疗储蓄账务的累积增额给付封顶，会保证较大的分摊份额流转进共同的 风险共保集团.

247. Insurers receive *risk-adjusted per capital payments* by the government and a separate flat rate premium from each insured person.

248. 保险公司从政府手中获得 人均风险调整付款，并且从每个参保者手中获得一份均等费率保险费.

249. Alert stewardship is needed to prevent the *capture* of such schemes by *lower risk*, better-off *groups*. (*)

250. 需要用警觉的管理工作来防止这些方案 争夺 经济状况较好的 低风险人群. (*)

251. *Risk pooling* strategies in each country need to be designed to increase such cross-subsidies.

252. 各国需要制定 风险共保 策略，以便增加这种交叉补贴.

253. Local and national *risk factors* need to be understood.

254. 需要了解地方的和全国的 危险因素.

255. Where there is no feasible organisational arrangement to boost pre-payment levels, both donors and governments should explore ways of building enabling mechanisms for the development or consolidation of large *risk pools.*

256. 凡没有提高预付水平的可行性组织安排的国家，捐赠者和政府都应开辟这样的途径，即创建能发展或强化大型 风险共保集团 的机制的途径.

257. In middle-income countries substantial mandatory, income and ***risk-based schemes*** often coexist.

258. 在中等收入国家常常同时还有大量收入和风险基础上的 强制性方案.

259. Statistical methods based on maximum likelihood estimation of the extended beta-binomial distribution have been developed to distinguish between variation across mothers in the number of children who have died due to chance and that due to differences in the ***underlying risks of death.*** (*)

260. 业已建立以扩展项式分布的最大偶然估计为基础的统计方法，   用于在母亲中区分死于意外事故和死于不同潜在死亡风险 的儿童在数量上的差异. (*)

261. The index presented in this table is meant to measure both fairness of financial contribution and ***financial risk protection;*** the basic concepts and principles are outlined in detail elsewhere.

262. 在这张表格中的指数意在衡量卫生经费资助的公正性和资助风险保护；基本概念和原则在别处详细阐述.

263. The index therefore reflects inequality in household financial contribution but particularly reflects those households ***at risk of impoverishment*** from high levels of health expenditure.

264. 因此，这个指数反映了家庭资金捐助的不同等性，   而并非是专门反映那些因为高水平卫生支出 有贫困危险的家庭的.

BIBLIOGRAPHY

Cao, K.H., and J.A. Birchenall. 2013. Agricultural productivity, structural change, and economic growth in post-reform China. *Journal of Development Economics* 30 (104): 165–180.

Du, Y., and C. Yang. 2014. Demographic transition and labour market changes: Implications for economic development in China. *Journal of Economic Surveys* 28 (4): 617–635.

Liu, X.B. 2013. Bibliometric analysis of the Republic of China literature based on CNKI database. *New Century Library* 8: 008.

Ma, R., L. Huang, D. Zhao, and L. Xu. 2015. Commercial health insurance–a new power to push china healthcare reform forward? *Value in Health* 18 (3): A103.

On the establishment of the basic healthcare security system for urban and suburban employees, State Council of the People's Republic of China, 14 December 1998. Original Chinese legislation available at http://www.gov.cn/banshi/2005-08/04/content_20256.htm.

Shen, J.J., S. Zhou, L. Xu, J. Chen, C.R. Cochran, and E.R. Fisher. 2014. Effects of the new health care reform on hospital performance in China: a seven-year trend from 2005 to 2011. *Journal of Health Care Finance* 41 (1): 0001.

© The Editor(s) (if applicable) and The Author(s) 2017
M. Ji, *Translation and Health Risk Knowledge Building in China,*
DOI 10.1007/978-981-10-4681-0

INDEX

© The Editor(s) (if applicable) and The Author(s) 2017
M. Ji, *Translation and Health Risk Knowledge Building in China*,
DOI 10.1007/978-981-10-4681-0